Oliver J. Morgan
Cheryl H. Litzke
Editors

Family Intervention in Substance Abuse: Current Best Practices

Family Intervention in Substance Abuse: Current Best Practices has been co-published simultaneously as *Alcoholism Treatment Quarterly*, Volume 26, Numbers 1/2 2008.

Pre-publication
REVIEWS,
COMMENTARIES,
EVALUATIONS . . .

"THIS BOOK BELONGS IN THE LIBRARY OF EVERY THERAPIST– it is timely, succinct, and practical; I will consider it required reading for my supervisees."

Robert R. DeYoung, EdD, EdS, MA
Founder, Family Center
for Behavioral Health

D0082194

More pre-publication
REVIEWS, COMMENTARIES, EVALUATIONS . . .

"**O**liver Morgan and Cheryl Litzke have brought together some of the best minds in family therapy and have produced what is CERTAIN TO BECOME A STANDARD IN THE FIELD. The contributors . . . have presented a range of approaches and each provides practical case examples highlighting both theory and technique. The extensive research cited by each contributor guides the reader to further exploration of each of the techniques and schools of therapy represented. . . . A welcome addition to literature in the field and WILL PROVE INVALUABLE TO PRACTITIONERS, TEACHERS AND STUDENTS ALIKE."

Edward A. Pane, MBA
Certified Addictions Counselor,
Certified Clinical Supervisor,
President and Chief Executive Officer,
Serento Gardens: Alcoholism
and Drug Services, Hazleton, PA

The Haworth Press

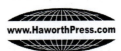
www.HaworthPress.com

Family Intervention in Substance Abuse: Current Best Practices

Family Intervention in Substance Abuse: Current Best Practices has been co-published simultaneously as *Alcoholism Treatment Quarterly*, Volume 26, Numbers 1/2 2008.

Monographic Separates from *Alcoholism Treatment Quarterly*®

For additional information on these and other Haworth Press titles, including descriptions, tables of contents, reviews, and prices, use the QuickSearch catalog at http://www.HaworthPress.com.

Family Intervention in Substance Abuse: Current Best Practices, edited by Oliver J. Morgan and Cheryl H. Litzke (Vol. 26, No. 1/2, 2008). *An examination of nine of the most current and evidence-based approaches to working with families that have an addicted or substance abusing member.*

Familial Responses to Alcohol Problems, edited by Judith L. Fischer, PhD, Miriam Mulsow, PhD, and Alan W. Korinek, PhD (Vol. 25, No. 1/2, 2007). *"Quality articles emphasizing a relational framework for understanding and treating substance abuse. . . . The life span findings from the Michigan Longitudinal study are particularly valuable for clinicians who see families both before and after substance abuse has been identified. . . . A strong addition to the libraries of experienced therapists and an excellent teaching tool for beginning therapists." (Marcia Lasswell, MS, Past President, American Association of Marriage and Family Therapy; Professor Emeritus, California State University, Pomona)*

Spirituality and Religiousness and Alcohol/Other Drug Problems: Treatment and Recovery Perspectives, edited by Brent B. Benda, PhD, and Thomas F. McGovern, EdD (Vol. 24, No. 1/2, 2006). *"Convincing evidence that spirituality and religiousness are not only relevant, but integral to our understanding the disease of addiction and the process of recovery." (Dr. Jeffry D. Roth, Editor, Journal of Groups in Addiction and Recovery; Author, Group Psychotherapy and Recovery from Addiction: Carrying the Message)*

Latinos and Alcohol Use/Abuse Revisited: Advances and Challenges for Prevention and Treatment Programs, edited by Melvin Delgado, PhD (Vol. 23, No. 2/3, 2005). *"For anyone interested in building a culturally competent system of care for Latinos, This book will provide invaluable guidance. . . . Fills a substantial gap in our knowledge about alcohol use and abuse among subgroups of Latinos. . . . Brings together research and practice knowledge on a broad range of topics, including the most recent trends in alcohol use and dependence among Latinos, service use and effectiveness, help-seeking behavior and barriers to treatment, the unmet needs of incarcerated Latinos, and ethnically sensitive interventions." (Carol Coohey, PhD, Associate Professor, University of Iowa School of Social Work)*

Responding to Physical and Sexual Abuse in Women with Alcohol and Other Drug and Mental Disorders: Program Building, edited by Bonita M. Veysey, PhD, and Colleen Clark, PhD (Vol. 22, No. 3/4, 2004). *"Highly recommended. Any clinician working with women (and their families) will appreciate the breadth and depth of this book and its use of clinical examples, treatment direction, and sobering statistics." (John Brick, PhD, MA, FAPA, Executive Director, Intoxikon International; Author of Drugs, the Brain, and Behavior and the Handbook of the Medical Consequences of Alcohol and Drug Abuse)*

Alcohol Problems in the United States: Twenty Years of Treatment Perspective, edited by Thomas F. McGovern, EdD, and William L. White, MA (Vol. 20, No. 3/4, 2002). *An overview of trends in the treatment of alcohol problems over a 20-year period.*

Homelessness Prevention in Treatment of Substance Abuse and Mental Illness: Logic Models and Implementation of Eight American Projects, edited by Kendon J. Conrad, PhD, Michael D. Matters, PhD, Patricia Hanrahan, and Daniel J. Luchins, MD (Vol. 17, No. 1/2, 1999). *Provides you with new insights into how you can help your clients overcome political, economic, and environmental barriers to treatment that can lead to homelessness.*

Alcohol Use/Abuse Among Latinos: Issues and Examples of Culturally Competent Services, edited by Melvin Delgado, PhD (Vol. 16, No. 1/2, 1998). *"This book will have widespread appeal for practitioners and educators involved in direct service delivery, organizational planning, research, or policy development." (Steven Lozano Applewhite, PhD, Associate Professor, Graduate School of Social Work, University of Houston, Texas)*

Treatment of the Addictions: Applications of Outcome Research for Clinical Management, edited by Norman S. Miller, MD (Vol. 12, No. 2, 1994). *"Ambitious and informative . . . Recommended to anybody involved in the practice of substance abuse treatment and research in treatment outcome." (The American Journal of Addictions)*

Self-Recovery: Treating Addictions Using Transcendental Meditation and Maharishi Ayur-Veda, edited by David F. O'Connell, PhD, and Charles N. Alexander, PhD (Vol. 11, No. 1/2/3/4, 1994). *"A scholarly trailblazer, a scientific first. . . . Those who work daily in the fight against substance abuse, violence, and illness will surely profit from reading this important volume. A valuable new tool in what may be America's most difficult battle." (Joseph Drew, PhD, Chair for Evaluation, Mayor's Advisory Committee on Drug Abuse, Washington, DC; Professor of Political Science, University of the District of Columbia)*

Treatment of the Chemically Dependent Homeless: Theory and Implementation in Fourteen American Projects, edited by Kendon J. Conrad, PhD, Cheryl I. Hultman, PhD, and John S. Lyons, PhD (Vol. 10, No. 3/4, 1993). *"A wealth of information and experience. . . . A very useful reference book for everyone seeking to develop their own treatment strategies with this patient group or the homeless mentally ill." (British Journal of Psychiatry)*

Treating Alcoholism and Drug Abuse Among Homeless Men and Women: Nine Community Demonstration Grants, edited by Milton Argeriou, PhD, and Dennis McCarty, PhD (Vol. 7, No. 1, 1990). *"Recommended to those in the process of trying to better serve chemically dependent homeless persons." (Journal of Psychoactive Drugs)*

Co-Dependency: Issues in Treatment and Recovery, edited by Bruce Carruth, PhD, and Warner Mendenhall, PhD (Vol. 6, No. 1, 1989). *"At last a book for clinicians that clearly defines co-dependency and gives helpful treatment approaches. Essential." (Margot Escott, MSW, Social Worker in Private Practice, Naples, Florida)*

The Treatment of Shame and Guilt in Alcoholism Counseling, edited by Ronald T. Potter-Efron, MSW, PhD, and Patricia S. Potter-Efron, MS, CACD III (Vol. 4, No. 2, 1989). *"Comprehensive in its coverage and provides important insights into the treatment of alcoholism, especially the importance to the recovery process of working through feelings of overwhelming shame and guilt. Recommended as required reading." (Australian Psychologist)*

Drunk Driving in America: Strategies and Approaches to Treatment, edited by Stephen K. Valle, ScD, CAC, FACATA (Vol. 3, No. 2, 1986). *Creative and thought-provoking methods related to research, policy, and treatment of the drunk driver.*

Alcohol Interventions: Historical and Sociocultural Approaches, edited by David L. Strug, PhD, S. Priyadarsini, PhD, and Merton M. Hyman (Supp. #1, 1986). *"A comprehensive and unique account of addictions treatment of centuries ago." (Federal Probation: A Journal of Correctional Philosophy)*

Treatment of Black Alcoholics, edited by Frances Larry Brisbane, PhD, MSW, and Maxine Womble, MA (Vol. 2, No. 3/4, 1985). *"Outstanding! In view of the paucity of research on the topic, this text presents some of the outstanding work done in this area." (Dr. Edward R. Smith, Department of Educational Psychology, University of Wisconsin-Milwaukee)*

Psychosocial Issues in the Treatment of Alcoholism, edited by David Cook, CSW, Christine Fewell, ACSW, and Shulamith Lala Ashenberg Straussner, DSW, CEAP (Vol. 2, No. 1, 1985). *"Well-written and informative; the topic areas are relevant to today's social issues and offer some new approaches to the treatment of alcoholics." (The American Journal of Occupational Therapy)*

Alcoholism and Sexual Dysfunction: Issues in Clinical Management, edited by David J. Powell, PhD (Vol. 1, No. 3, 1984). *"It does a good job of explicating the linkage between two of the most common health problems in the U.S. today." (Journal of Sex & Marital Therapy)*

Family Intervention in Substance Abuse: Current Best Practices

Oliver J. Morgan
Cheryl H. Litzke
Editors

Family Intervention in Substance Abuse: Current Best Practices has been co-published simultaneously as *Alcoholism Treatment Quarterly*, Volume 26, Numbers 1/2 2008.

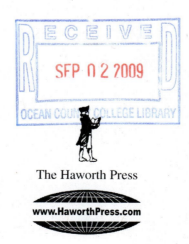

The Haworth Press

www.HaworthPress.com

Family Intervention in Substance Abuse: Current Best Practices has been co-published simultaneously as *Alcoholism Treatment Quarterly*, Volume 26, Numbers 1/2 2008.

The development, preparation, and publication of this work has been undertaken with great care. However, the publisher, employees, editors, and agents of The Haworth Press and all imprints of The Haworth Press, including The Haworth Medical Press® and Pharmaceutical Products Press®, are not responsible for any errors contained herein or for consequences that may ensue from use of materials or information contained in this work. With regard to case studies, identities and circumstances of individuals discussed herein have been changed to protect confidentiality. Any resemblance to actual persons, living or dead, is entirely coincidental.

The Haworth Press is committed to the dissemination of ideas and information according to the highest standards of intellectual freedom and the free exchange of ideas. Statements made and opinions expressed in this publication do not necessarily reflect the views of the Publisher, Directors, management, or staff of The Haworth Press, or an endorsement by them.

The Haworth Press, 10 Alice Street, Binghamton, 13904-1580 USA

Library of Congress Cataloging-in-Publication Data

Family intervention in substance abuse : current best practices / Oliver J. Morgan, Cheryl H. Litzke, editors.
    p. ; cm.
    "Co-published simultaneously as Alcoholism Treatment Quarterly, Volume 26, Numbers 1/2 2008."
    Includes bibliographical references and index.
    ISBN 978-0-7890-3757-2 (hard cover : alk. paper) – ISBN 978-0-7890-3758-9 (soft cover : alk. paper)
    1. Substance abuse–Treatment. 2. Alcoholism–Treatment. 3. Substance abuse–Patients–Family relationships. 4. Alcoholics–Family relationships. 5. Family psychotherapy. I. Morgan, Oliver J. II. Litzke, Cheryl H. III. Alcoholism treatment quarterly.
    [DNLM: 1. Substance-Related Disorders–therapy. 2. Evidence-Based Medicine. 3. Family–psychology. 4. Family Therapy–methods. 5. Models, Psychological. 6. Motivation. W1 AL3147 v.27 no.1/2 2008 / WM 270 F19755 2008]

RC564.F34 2008
362.29–dc22

2007031310

This section provides you with a list of major indexing & abstracting services and other tools for bibliographic access. That is to say, each service began covering this periodical during the year noted in the right column. Most Websites which are listed below have indicated that they will either post, disseminate, compile, archive, cite or alert their own Website users with research-based content from this work. (This list is as current as the copyright date of this publication.)

<u>Abstracting, Website/Indexing Coverage</u> . . . . <u>Year When Coverage Began</u>

- *Abstracts in Anthropology <http://www.baywood.com/ Journals/PreviewJournals.asp?Id=0001-3455>* **1991**
- *Academic Search Premier (EBSCO) <http://search.ebscohost.com>* **1995**
- *Academic Search Alumni Edition (EBSCO) <http://search.ebscohost.com>* **2007**
- *Academic Search Complete (EBSCO) <http://search.ebscohost.com>* **2006**
- *Academic Search Elite (EBSCO) <http://search.ebscohost.com>* . . . **1995**
- *Academic Source Premier (EBSCO) <http://search.ebscohost.com>* **2006**
- *Addiction Abstracts (Published in collaboration with the National Addiction Centre & Carfax, Taylor & Francis) <http://www.tandf.co.uk/addiction-abs>* **1995**
- *Alcohol Studies Database <http://cf7-test.scc-net.rutgers.edu/ alcohol_studies/alcohol/index.htm>* **2007**
- *ATForum.com <http://www.atforum.com>* **2006**
- *British Library Inside (The British Library) <http://www.bl.uk/services/current/inside.html>* **2006**
- *Cambridge Scientific Abstracts (ProQuest CSA) <http://www.csa.com>* **2006**
- *Child Development Abstracts (Taylor & Francis) <shttp://www.tandf.co.uk>* **2007**

(continued)

(continued)

(continued)

Bibliographic Access

Special Bibliographic Notes related to special journal issues (separates) and indexing/abstracting:

- indexing/abstracting services in this list will also cover material in any "separate" that is co-published simultaneously with Haworth's special thematic journal issue or DocuSerial. Indexing/abstracting usually covers material at the article/chapter level.
- monographic co-editions are intended for either non-subscribers or libraries which intend to purchase a second copy for their circulating collections.
- monographic co-editions are reported to all jobbers/wholesalers/approval plans. The source journal is listed as the "series" to assist the prevention of duplicate purchasing in the same manner utilized for books-in-series.
- to facilitate user/access services all indexing/abstracting services are encouraged to utilize the co-indexing entry note indicated at the bottom of the first page of each article/chapter/contribution.
- this is intended to assist a library user of any reference tool (whether print, electronic, online, or CD-ROM) to locate the monographic version if the library has purchased this version but not a subscription to the source journal.
- individual articles/chapters in any Haworth publication are also available through the Haworth Document Delivery Service (HDDS).

AS PART OF OUR CONTINUING COMMITMENT TO BETTER SERVE OUR LIBRARY PATRONS, WE ARE PROUD TO BE WORKING WITH THE FOLLOWING ELECTRONIC SERVICES:

AGGREGATOR SERVICES

- *EBSCOhost*   - *Ingenta*   - *J-Gate*   - *Minerva*
- *OCLC FirstSearch*   - *Oxmill*   - *SwetsWise*

LINK RESOLVER SERVICES

- *1Cate (Openly Informatics)*   - *ChemPort (American Chemical Society)*
- *CrossRef*   - *Gold Rush (Coalliance)*   - *LinkOut (PubMed)*
- *LINKplus (Atypon)*   *LinkSolver (Ovid)*   - *LinkSource with A-to-Z (EBSCO)*
- *Resource Linker (Ulrich's)*   - *SerialsSolutions (ProQuest)*   - *SFX (Ex Libris)*
- *Sirsi Resolver (SirsiDynix)*   - *Tour (TDnet)*   - *Vlink (Extensity)*
- *WebBridge (Innovative Interfaces)*

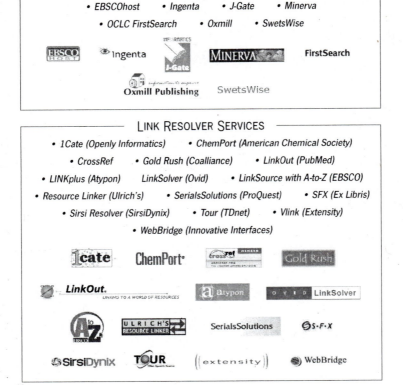

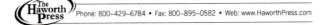
The Haworth Press Phone: 800–429–6784 • Fax: 800–895–0582 • Web: www.HaworthPress.com

Family Intervention in Substance Abuse: Current Best Practices

CONTENTS

ABOUT THE EDITORS

Oliver J. Morgan, PhD, is Professor and Chair of the Department of Counseling and Human Services at the University of Scranton, Scranton, Pennsylvania. He is a National Certified Counselor (NCC) and licensed Marriage and Family Therapist (LMFT), as well as an Approved Supervisor with the American Association for Marriage and Family Therapy. He has published a number of articles in the area of addiction studies and his co-edited book, *Addiction and Spirituality: A Multidisciplinary Approach* (1999) has been well received. He is on the Steering Committee for the Institute for Research, Education and Training in Addictions (IRETA), which sponsors the Northeast Addiction Technology Transfer Center (NeATTC), and was recently appointed to the Board of the Guest House Institute.

Cheryl H. Litzke, PhD (Cand.), is Clinical Assistant Professor in the Programs in Couple and Family Therapy, College of Nursing and Health Professions, at Drexel University, Philadelphia, Pennsylvania. She is a licensed Marriage and Family Therapist (LMFT), Clinical Member and Approved Supervisor with the American Association for Marriage and Family Therapy (AAMFT).

Introduction

Oliver J. Morgan
Cheryl H. Litzke

Not so long ago, when a concerned family member called for help with a drinking or drug-using loved one, most of us as practitioners had few good options available.

We could suggest some version of an "intervention" popularized by the Johnson Institute (Johnson, 1973, 1986), but family members were often unwilling or unable to follow through with the secret planning and ultimate confrontation this model required. Further, although currently in vogue, as seen in the television show "Intervention" on the Arts & Entertainment channel, the success rate of this clinical strategy is actually quite low. According to Stanton (2004), who reviews the available outcome studies of intervention methods, the success rate ranges from 0-36% (p. 170). The average across available studies is actually 20%, or only one person in every five. And, even if the model is fully deployed, the addicted loved one often finds ingenious ways to circumvent the process. The inevitable return to abuse, then, is demoralizing for all concerned (Dundas, 2006).

Of course, we could always suggest the Al-Anon route (White & Savage, 2005), but this too had its drawbacks. Families did not want to abandon their loved ones to their own devices. They were not willing to "detach with love," if this meant putting their addict at extreme risk. They actually wanted to *help*, despite our pious warnings about the

[Haworth co-indexing entry note]: "Introduction." Morgan, Oliver, J., and Cheryl H. Litzke. Co-published simultaneously in *Alcoholism Treatment Quarterly* (The Haworth Press) Vol. 26, No. 1/2, 2008, pp. 1-8; and: *Family Intervention in Substance Abuse: Current Best Practices* (ed: Oliver J. Morgan, and Cheryl H. Litzke) The Haworth Press, 2008, pp. 1-8. Single or multiple copies of this article are available for a fee from The Haworth Document Delivery Service [1-800-HAWORTH, 9:00 a.m. - 5:00 p.m. (EST). E-mail address: docdelivery@haworthpress.com].

dangers of "enabling." Concerned family members wanted to do something effective, but we often did not have useful strategies to offer.

To be honest, many practitioners really believed that sobriety was something of a crap-shoot for these families as well as for the person with alcohol and other drug problems. Unfortunately, this belief was reinforced by many in the addiction treatment and recovery communities, and abetted by the lack of hope among individual and family therapists. "If and when the addict suffers enough," these professionals would tell us, "then there may be a chance. But, he or she must first 'hit bottom.' Families should get out of the way and stop trying to be helpful. They only make things worse. And, by the way, family members are likely as sick as the addict." In order to confirm this last assertion, many addiction practitioners were willing to label as "co-alcoholics," or "enablers," or "co-dependents" any family members who were unwilling to follow through with therapeutic suggestions or who balked at these gloomy predictions (see White & Savage, 2005).

It was not a pretty picture, and families often intuited our sense of frustration and hopelessness about these cases. Within the field of family therapy, however, some powerful alternative ways of thinking and intervening were being explored in dialogue with family systems perspectives and behavioral techniques, but these never quite seemed to make it into the mainstream, either of the family therapy literature or of the best practices in addiction studies. The works of Steinglass (1987) and Berenson (1976a & b), of Bepko and Krestan (1985, 1990), of Stanton (1982) and Kaufman (1985), of McCrady (1989) and Treadway (1989), to name a few, were acknowledged but not widely accepted or fully implemented. Instead a truncated "family therapy" view was imported into addiction treatment (see, for example, Beattie, 1987; Kitchens, 1991; Wegscheider, 1981; Woititz, 1983), and important systems thinking was by-passed.

As practicing family therapists and clinical educators with strong interests in addiction studies and treatment, we have been puzzled by these developments. Addiction treatment facilities and counselors still seem to operate as though families with an addicted member are troublesome at best and not worth more than a few meetings within a "comprehensive" treatment plan for individual addicts. Family therapists often seem not well informed about the current "best practices" within their own field for working with alcohol and drug-affected clients and their families. This is contrasted with the findings in recent surveys revealing that 84% to 88% of marriage and family therapists actually treat clients with alcohol-related problems (Northey, 2002; Roberts &

McCrady, 2003). Only recently has there been a movement toward collaboration between the addiction and family therapy establishments (Center for Substance Abuse Treatment, 2004).[1] Now it seems may be the time for further work linking these two approaches.

In editing this volume, we hope to make widely available a selection of the most powerful treatment approaches developed at the interface of addiction studies and family therapy. Indeed a series of contemporary outcome studies identifies many of these approaches as the most promising and effective tools in our current clinical arsenal (Stanton, 2004; Liddle & Dakof, 1995; Edwards & Steinglass, 1995; Rotunda & O'Farrell, 1997; Rotunda, Scherer & Imm, 1995). It seems clear at this juncture that family-based understandings and approaches for substance abuse must be taken more seriously within both the addiction and family therapy treatment communities.

The chapters within this volume provide a firm and effective foundation for family-based work with substance abuse and addiction. We asked the contributors to this volume–teams of clinician-researchers who have developed promising approaches to the problem–to compose essays describing their work with substance abuse and families. We asked them to provide both the theory underneath their practice and models for practical application. We asked them to write specifically for "research-savvy practitioners." Each chapter accomplishes these tasks, while also providing outcome data for evaluation by our readers and a good sense of where to go to acquire more information on any particular approach. As Editors we are grateful for the clarity and professionalism provided by each (team of) contributor(s).

This publication is laid out, then, in three segments. First there is the "Introduction" to set the stage for the main articles to come. It has a companion piece at the end: David Treadway's Practitioner's Response entitled, "Grace Happens." David has added to his now classic work in the field of addiction and family therapy, *Before it's too late* (1989), several more personal and literary works (2004, 1996) that emanate from his clinical practice and exploration. His creative and exploratory streak is again in evidence in his appreciative essay at the end of this collection. We are grateful for his contribution and support throughout this project.

The two main sections of this publication, Family Systems Models and Evidence-Based Models, are divided up somewhat arbitrarily but with a few purposes in mind. Most of the approaches in this collection are based on a fundamental understanding of "family systems." Individuals are seen as embedded within a network of dynamic relationships.

Changing destructive symptoms, such as alcohol and other drug problems, is understood to occur through altering the patterns and structures of these relationships. This is the heart of clinical systems thinking. A variety of contingency management and behavioral techniques have been integrated as tools for this change.

Some of the approaches have more extensive effectiveness and outcome research behind them. These are the Evidence-Based Models. The Family Systems Models included in this collection tilt more in the direction of straightforward systems thinking, enhanced by inclusion of more contemporary addiction approaches, such as motivational interviewing, stages of change, and relapse prevention.

Section I contains three samplings of these Family Systems Models. Peter Steinglass, a long-standing champion of family therapeutic work with alcohol and other drug problems, begins with a review of some history surrounding substance abuse and family therapy treatment and then looks deeply into the questions raised by more contemporary approaches. In particular his more recent combination of motivational interviewing with empirically-grounded family systems thinking is an exciting development. We are delighted to be one of the first venues in which Peter has published this new integration.

In *Beyond "Happily Ever After,"* Joyce Schmid and Stephanie Brown present their model from the Family Recovery Project, integrating family systems within a developmental recovery perspective. The joining of this approach with a dynamic Twelve Step perspective is one of its strengths. Their presentation–an extended case discussion and analysis– allows readers to see the operation of many different elements within the progression of recovery stages.

Liepman, Flachier and Tareen's contribution on *Family Behavior Loop Mapping* provides a fascinating view into the integration of systems thinking with cognitive and behavioral assessment and interventions. From the beginning allusion to Dr. Jekyll and Mr. Hyde as a metaphor for the experience of alcohol and other drug problems to the final suggestions of exploring similar dynamics in other episodic or recurring illnesses, this will be a challenging and informative chapter for all readers of this volume.

An important insight provided by all these approaches highlights what many clinicians have come to understand, namely, that we must attend to the differences between the "dry" and "wet" states that oscillate in these troubled families. When we come to understand both the losses AND the benefits brought on by the use of alcohol and other drugs for these individuals and families, we will be able to provide much more effective help.

Section II on Evidence-Based Models presents a number of family therapy approaches that are receiving high praise for effectiveness in recent outcome studies. Again using an extended clinical case, Briones and his colleagues in the *Brief Strategic Family Therapy* (BSFT) school present a very effective model for helping families with alcohol and other drug abusing children and adolescents. Attending to the already-known basics of family structure, communication, and the quality of family relationships, this approach can demonstrate marked improvements, not only in treating alcohol and other drug problems but in a host of other adolescent difficulties, such as underachievement, delinquency, and risky sexual behavior.

This approach shares many similar treatment goals and some similar clinical thinking with two other models presented in this section. Rowe and Liddle present *Multidimensional Family Therapy* (MDFT), a family-based approach which integrates current knowledge about risk and protective factors for teen alcohol abuse and relapse patterns. Sheidow and Henggeler present *Multisystemic Therapy* (MST), which has demonstrated effectiveness not only with alcohol and other drug abusing adolescents but with delinquents as well.

Interestingly, these three approaches in particular–BSFT, MDFT and MST–have demonstrated their effectiveness in several different treatment settings, including home-based family work. They intentionally attempt to include sensitivity to cultural difference in their work, and focus on improving the full range of family relationships and structures as the path to ameliorating troublesome adolescent behaviors. Not only can they demonstrate change in troublesome symptoms, but they improve overall family functioning as well.

The *ARISE Model*, presented by Landau and Garrett, is a therapeutic approach specifically designed to increase the effectiveness of engaging alcohol and other drug abusers into treatment. It utilizes an approach, implemented by families, built around a process for changing the system of rewards around alcohol and other drug use–and non-use–over time and leads ultimately to an "invitational [vs. a confrontational] intervention." Supporting sober behavior and discouraging drinking behavior is also the focus of the *CRAFT Model*, presented by Jane Ellen Smith, Robert Meyers, and Julia Austin. This approach, which again provides families with the tools to influence positively the drinking or drug use of a loved one, also helps family members to increase their own well-being while working to achieve sobriety within the family. It was recently presented as a state-of-the-art treatment approach in the televised HBO series on *Addiction* (see website at http://www.hbo.com/addiction/).

Finally, O'Farrell and Fals-Stewart give us a fascinating look into their work with couples struggling with alcohol and other drug problems. *Behavioral Couples Therapy* (BCT) integrates couples work with behavioral techniques, judicious use of recovery-based medications (e.g., disulfiram, naltrexone), individual and group counseling, and Twelve Step work. It has a proven track record of success with these difficult problems, and the techniques used can help all practitioners working with these difficulties.

We are grateful to all those who submitted and revised manuscripts for this project. They have made a significant contribution to the state of our knowledge in this important field of family therapy and addiction studies. We are grateful to those who worked with us as readers, including Paul Henry, Thomas Collins, and Elizabeth Jacob. A special "thank you" is owed to Dr. Tom McGovern, General Editor of *Alcoholism Treatment Quarterly*, who believed in this project from the outset and supported it from beginning to end.

Finally, we, as Editors, would like to acknowledge the work of Dr. Loretta Sylvia of Wake Forest University, one of our contributors, who succumbed to a deadly cancer in Fall of 2006. The chapter on *Family Behavior Loop Mapping* is dedicated to her. We both also lost a valued teacher and mentor during the time of this project: Dr. Ivan Boszormenyi-Nagy. Ivan impressed on us the value of relationships, mutuality, and care, not only on overall health, but on achieving success in altering destructive patterns in persons' lives. He taught us hope. This is a critically important virtue in the healing of relationships damaged by abuse of alcohol and other drugs.

We hope this collection provides readers with a cause for hope, and the tools to make it come alive.

NOTE

1. A recent collaborative publication between the National Institute on Alcohol Abuse and Alcoholism (NIAAA), the Alcohol Research to Practice Network, and the American Association for Marriage and Family Therapy (AAMFT) signaled this new movement. Roberts and McCrady's Guide, *Alcohol problems in intimate relationships: Identification and intervention* (February 2003) is available from NIAAA, AAMFT or online at http://pubs.niaaa.nih.gov/publications/niaaa-guide/index.htm.

REFERENCES

Beattie, M. (1987). *Codependent No More: How to Stop Controlling Others and Start Caring for Yourself.* New York, NY: Harper & Row.

Bepko, C., & Krestan, J. A. (1990). *Too Good for Her Own Good: Breaking Free from the Burden of Female Responsibility.* New York, NY: Harper & Row.

Bepko, C., & Krestan, J. A. (1985). *The Responsibility Trap: A Blueprint for Treating the Alcoholic Family.* New York, NY: Free Press.

Berenson, D. (1976a). A family approach to alcoholism. *Psychiatric Opinion, 13,* 33-38.

Berenson, D. (1976b). Alcohol and the family system. In P. Guerin (Ed.), *Family therapy: Theory and practice* (pp. 284-297). New York, NY: Gardner Press.

Center for Substance Abuse Treatment. (2004). *Substance Abuse Treatment and Family Therapy.* Treatment Improvement Protocol (TIP) Series, No. 39. DHHS Publication No. (SMA) 04-3957. Rockville, MD: Substance Abuse and Mental Health Services Administration.

Dundas, I. (2006). The dilemma of confrontation: Coping with problem drinking in the family. *Alcoholism Treatment Quarterly, 24*(4), 79-98.

Edwards, M. E., & Steinglass, P. (1995). Family therapy treatment outcomes for alcoholism. *Journal of Marital and Family Therapy, 21,* 475-509.

Johnson, V. E. (1973). *I'll Quit Tomorrow.* New York, NY: Harper & Row.

Johnson, V. E. (1986). *Intervention: How to Help Those Who Don't Want Help.* Minneapolis, MN: Johnson Institute.

Kaufman, E. (1985). *Substance Abuse and Family Therapy.* Orlando, FL: Grune & Stratton.

Kitchens, J. A. (1991). *Understanding and Treating Codependence.* Englewood Cliffs, NJ: Prentice Hall.

Liddle, H. A., & Dakof, G. A. (1995). Efficacy of family therapy for drug abuse: Promising but not definitive. *Journal of Marital and Family Therapy, 21,* 511-543.

McCrady, B. S. (1989). Outcomes of family-involved alcoholism treatment. In M. Galanter (Ed.), *Recent developments in alcoholism, Volume VII: Treatment issues* (pp. 165-182). New York, NY: Plenum.

Northey, W. F. (2002). Characteristics and clinical practices of marriage and family therapists: A national survey. *Journal of Marital and Family Therapy, 28*(4), 487-494.

Roberts, L. J., & McCrady, B. S. (February 2003). *Alcohol problems in intimate relationships: Identification and intervention: A Guide for Marriage and Family Therapists.* Washington, DC: NIAAA, NIH. [NIH Publication No. 03-5284].

Rotunda, R. J., & O'Farrell, T. J. (1997). Marital and family therapy of alcohol use disorders: Bridging the gap between research and practice. *Professional Psychology: Research and Practice, 28*(3), 246-252.

Rotunda, R. J., Scherer, D. G., & Imm, P. S. (1995). Family systems and alcohol misuse: Research on the effects of alcoholism on family functioning and effective family interventions. *Professional Psychology: Research and Practice, 26*(1), 95-104.

Stanton, M. D. (2004). Getting reluctant substance abusers to engage in treatment/self-help: A review of outcomes and clinical options. *Journal of Marital and Family therapy, 30*(2), 165-182.

Stanton, M. D., Todd, T. C., & Associates. (1982). *The Family Therapy of Drug Abuse and Addiction.* New York, NY: Guilford.

Steinglass, P., Bennett, L. A., Wolin, S. J., & Reiss, D. (1987). *The Alcoholic Family.* New York, NY: Basic.

Treadway, D. C. (2004). *Intimacy, Change, and Other Therapeutic Mysteries: Stories of Clinicians and Clients.* New York, NY: Guilford.

Treadway, D. C. (1996). *Dead Reckoning: A Therapist Confronts His Own Grief.* New York, NY: Basic Books.

Treadway, D. C. (1989). *Before It's Too Late: Working with Substance Abuse in the Family.* New York, NY: W.W. Norton.

Wegscheider, S. (1981). *Another Chance: Hope and Health for Alcoholic Families.* New York, NY: Science and Behavior Books.

White, W., & Savage, B. (2005). All in the family: Alcohol and other drug problems, recovery, advocacy. *Alcoholism Treatment Quarterly, 23*(4), 3-37.

Woititz, J. G. (1983). *Adult Children of Alcoholics.* Deerfield Beach, FL: Health Communications, Inc.

doi:10.1300/J020v26n01_01

Family Systems
and Motivational Interviewing:
A Systemic-Motivational Model
for Treatment of Alcohol
and Other Drug Problems

Peter Steinglass, MD

SUMMARY. Despite growing evidence of the impact of substance abuse disorders on families and the effectiveness of family-based treatment approaches for these disorders, family therapy remains an underutilized modality for these conditions. One reason may be the relative paucity of treatment models combining family systems concepts with current

---

Peter Steinglass is Director of the Center for Substance Abuse and the Family at the Ackerman Institute for the Family, 149 East 78th Street, New York City, NY 10021.

[Haworth co-indexing entry note]: "Family Systems and Motivational Interviewing: A Systemic-Motivational Model for Treatment of Alcohol and Other Drug Problems." Steinglass, Peter. Co-published simultaneously in *Alcoholism Treatment Quarterly* (The Haworth Press) Vol. 26, No. 1/2, 2008, pp. 9-29; and: *Family Intervention in Substance Abuse: Current Best Practices* (ed: Oliver J. Morgan, and Cheryl H. Litzke) The Haworth Press, 2008, pp. 9-29. Single or multiple copies of this article are available for a fee from The Haworth Document Delivery Service [1-800-HAWORTH, 9:00 a.m. - 5:00 p.m. (EST). E-mail address: docdelivery@haworthpress.com].

Available online at http://atq.haworthpress.com
doi:10.1300/J020v26n01_02

advances in substance abuse treatment. This paper describes one such approach, called the Systemic Motivational Model, a treatment model that has as its goal the integration of the empirically-grounded family systems model of alcoholism treatment first developed in the 1980s (the Family Life History model) with the core ideas encompassed in Motivational Enhancement Therapy. doi:10.1300/J020v26n01_02 *[Article copies available for a fee from The Haworth Document Delivery Service: 1-800-HAWORTH. E-mail address: <docdelivery@haworthpress.com> Website: <http://www.HaworthPress.com> © 2008 by The Haworth Press. All rights reserved.]*

KEYWORDS. Alcoholism treatment, family therapy, motivational interviewing, transtheoretical model, alcohol-other drug problems, families

INTRODUCTION

The past three decades have witnessed a growing body of research and clinical data establishing not only that family factors play a significant role in the onset and course of chronic alcoholism, but also that the challenges to family life of alcohol abuse are multiple and substantial, including family violence, sexual abuse of children, financial crises, and so forth (Baucom et al., 1998; Rotunda & O'Farrell, 1997; Rotunda, Scherer, & Imm, 1995; Velleman, 2006). These data, in turn, have been cited as supporting a position that effective treatment for alcoholism needs to target the needs of all family members.

This view has been further reinforced by the growing evidence that family-focused treatment approaches to alcohol abuse and dependence both significantly increase engagement and retention of the alcoholic individual in treatment, and improve treatment outcomes for all involved (Edwards & Steinglass, 1995; Miller, Meyers, & Tonigan, 1999; O'Farrell & Fals-Stewart, 2002; Stanton & Heath, 2005; Thomas & Corcoran, 2001). Yet despite this evidence, it is still the case that family approaches to alcoholism treatment are at best a minor part of most residential and ambulatory treatment programs.

A number of factors have contributed to this marginalization of family-focused treatment approaches to alcoholism. At the top of the list are health care systems built around the diagnosis and treatment of individuals, and health insurance policies that often exclude reimbursement for couples and family therapy. But equally important is the minimal training that addiction professionals receive in family systems assessment and treatment, and the parallel paucity of attention paid to substance abuse issues in most marital and family therapy graduate training programs.

As a consequence, most substance abuse therapists are only peripherally aware of the advances made in family therapy approaches to alcoholism treatment, and most family therapists still think of substance abuse treatment as limited to individual therapy, pharmacotherapy, and self-help groups. Given this situation, there would appear to be ample room for an exploration of integrative approaches that bring together some of the newer ideas in family therapy, on the one hand, and substance abuse treatment, on the other.

In this paper I will be describing one such approach, a model that has as its goal the integration of a family systems model of alcoholism I first described in the 1980s (Steinglass et al., 1987) with the core ideas encompassed in the motivational interviewing approach to alcoholism treatment that have emerged during the 1990s and to the present (Miller & Rollnick, 2002). The family systems model of alcoholism, which we called the Family Life History (FLH) model (Steinglass, 1980), was based on empirical research findings emerging from a series of studies of families with alcoholic members (Bennett et al., 1987; Steinglass, Davis & Berenson, 1977; Steinglass, 1981). Motivational Interviewing (MI), on the other hand, has been seen primarily as a set of techniques applicable for therapeutic work with individuals, and has been closely associated with the newer ideas to addictions treatment encompassed in harm reduction and relapse prevention approaches to therapy (Marlatt & Gordon, 1985; Marlatt & Tapert, 1993; Marlatt, 1998). It is the confluence of these ideas that underlie the approach to addictions treatment called Motivational Enhancement Therapy (MET) (Miller et al., 1992).

Many of us who have argued for the greater use of family-focused treatment interventions for alcoholism have been impressed by three sets of research findings supportive of a family therapy perspective–first, that the active inclusion of family members during the assessment/ diagnostic phase of treatment substantially increases the clarity of the clinical picture (i.e., quantity/frequency of drinking behavior and its impact on family, work, social relationships, and physical health), second, that family involvement early on increases subsequent engagement of *both* the patient *and* family in on-going treatment (including rehabilitation and aftercare phases of treatment), and third, that all these approaches substantially improve long-term outcomes not only for the alcoholic family member (e.g., increased sobriety rates), but for others in the family as well (e.g., increased marital satisfaction and stability).

These findings have come largely from effectiveness and efficacy studies of three types of treatment approaches–behavioral family therapy models (Lipps, 1999; O'Farrell, Choquette, & Cutter, 1998; Rotunda, Scherer & Imm, 1995), network therapy models (Galanter, 1999; Garrett et al., 1997; Landau et al., 2004), and motivational enhancement models (Meyers et al., 1999). As such, they are approaches that either extend classical conditioning principles to interactional behavior with particular emphasis on the interactional contingencies that contribute to alcohol use, or use the substance user's social and family networks to help support behavior change. Thus although they are therapies that involve family members actively in treatment, the target for treatment remains the individual who is abusing alcohol.

Our family systems model, on the other hand, conceptualizes *the family itself* as the primary treatment target.[1] This is based on the notion that many families who have lived with chronic alcoholism in their midst over long periods of time evolve into what has been called *alcoholic systems* meaning systems in which important components of family life have been structured and shaped primarily by the family's responses to the challenges attendant to alcohol abuse and its effect on interactional behavior within the family. And in addition to this more radical position of seeing the family rather than the individual as the patient, family systems treatment models also emphasize three additional components as critical to the therapy approach:

- a therapeutic stance that emphasizes *therapist neutrality*, the use of *non-pathologizing language* with patients and families, and *family-therapist collaboration* (rather than a hierarchical approach in which the therapist takes the position of "expert" and unilaterally defines the treatment goals for the family);
- a conviction that central to the success of treatment is the ability to ascertain both *individual and family-level beliefs* about the role of alcohol use in family life; and
- a conviction that therapy, to be effective, must include a credible *action plan* for addressing the drinking behavior itself that is *embraced by the entire family*.

As I will point out later in the paper, each of the above components parallels similar concepts that are central to ideas put forward in motivational interviewing. It is for this reason that an approach to alcoholism treatment that combines family systems and MI concepts has been so appealing. In addition, by drawing on these parallels, one can develop a treatment model that also potentially bridges the divide currently separating the worlds of family therapy and substance abuse treatment. That is, the potential synergy encompassed in family systems ideas and MI also means that both family therapists and addiction specialists can see their core ideas represented in a systemic-motivational approach to alcoholism treatment.

I will develop this argument by reviewing the main components of the systemic-motivation model as they developed chronologically. First I will summarize the research experiences that led to the FLH model and the treatment approach based on this model. Then I will discuss some of the limitations we experienced in applying the treatment approach. And finally, I will discuss how the ideas encompassed in MI and the harm reduction approach to alcoholism treatment, when married to the family systems ideas in the FLH model, offer significant potential advantages in a next generation family-focused treatment model.

BACKGROUND
FOR THE SYSTEMIC-MOTIVATIONAL MODEL

The Family Life History Model: During the 1970s, my colleagues and I carried out a series of studies of families with alcoholic members who were observed in laboratory and home settings. Because we were able to observe these families both during periods of time when alcohol was and was not being consumed, we were able to contrast patterns of family interaction in the presence versus absence of active drinking (Steinglass, Davis, & Berenson, 1977). Three types of measures were used in these studies: (a) home observations utilizing a formal coding system to track family use of time and space in the home (Steinglass, 1979); (b) detailed family interviews to trace the relationship between alcohol use and family rituals (Wolin, Bennett & Noonan, 1980); and (c) a laboratory-based interactional problem-solving task (Reiss et al., 1980).

Two major propositions emerged from these studies—first, that the families we were observing had two very different and distinctive interactional styles depending on whether they were in the "alcohol-on" or "alcohol-off" state; and second, that in many instances family behaviors exhibited during the "alcohol-on" periods seemed to have adaptive, problem-solving capabilities (that is, were it not for the fact that they were occurring in conjunction with excessive alcohol use). Further, this picture of life in these families as cycling back and forth between these two different interactional states tied to the presence or absence of alcohol also seemed to be a major contributory factor to the behavioral rigidity that was one of the cardinal features of these families. Put another way, we came to see these families as *alcoholic systems* in that alcoholism and alcohol-related behaviors had assumed the status of a central organizing principle for family life (analogous to the way in which other families might identify themselves as "child-centered" or "work-centered" families).

A major therapeutic implication of this work was the need to consider both the adaptive as well as disruptive aspects of alcohol abuse on family life as a critical initial step in the treatment process. In particular, it suggested that attempts to "remove alcohol" from the family (by placing the alcoholic family member in a traditional abstinence-oriented, rehabilitation program) could easily disrupt the delicate homeostatic balance existing in the family, with unpredictable sequelae.

But also implied in this work was the potential usefulness of the measurement techniques used in the research studies as clinical tools for family assessment. Would it be possible, for example, to develop interview protocols for examining a family's daily routines, family rituals, and short-term problem-solving strategies, and to track how changes in behavior were tied to on-off alcohol use? Because the answer was yes, one important clinical contribution of these early studies was to suggest a framework for assessment in working with families in which chronic alcoholism was a major issue.

The second step in the overall development of our clinical model was to place the core ideas emerging from our initial studies within a *developmental context*. How might we conceptualize the process leading to the family's organization around alcohol that was the striking end step we were observing in our earlier studies? Why would families seemingly choose a life path that to the outside observer had such negative consequences?

Earlier speculations had focused on family pathology as the explanation, that is, that the needs of one or more family members led to collusion with the alcoholic family member in the initiation and perpetuation of abusive drinking behavior. Our view, instead, was that the more frequent situation entailed a multi-step process of accommodation on the part of the family to the drinker and his or her needs associated with worsening alcohol abuse.

Focusing on the same three areas of family life mentioned above–family routines, family rituals, and family problem-solving strategies–we were able to track a process in which the family gradually restructured its life to accommodate to the demands of alcohol abuse by altering its patterns of daily life, by allowing important family rituals like holidays and vacations to be disrupted because of alcohol-related demands, and by delaying important family decisions when active drinking was occurring (see Figure 1).

We used the metaphor of *invasion* to describe this process–that alcohol was invading these important aspects of family life. The consequence, we proposed, was a *distortion* of the usual trajectory of development of the family system. The end product (as noted above) was a behavioral system in which alcoholism had become the *central organizing principle* of family life. And once again, the therapeutic implication was that treatment directed primarily at the alcoholic individual was misguided. Instead, a family systems treatment approach seemed called for whenever one was dealing with the type of situation described above.

FIGURE 1. Steps in the Process of Family Organization Around Substance Abuse.

Impact of Alcohol/Substance Abuse on Families

Accommodation to Alcohol/Drug Needs
↓
Restructuring of Family Routines
↓
Delayed Decision-Making
↓
Imbalance in Resource Distribution
↓
Invasion/Disruption of Family Rituals
↓
Distortion of Family Identity
↓
Alcoholism/Drug Abuse as Central Organizing Principle

The Alcoholic Family Treatment Model: Using the FLH model of alcohol and the family, a four-stage treatment model was developed (outlined in Table 1) which included the familiar components of assessment, detoxification, relapse prevention, and rehabilitation but this time with each of these components addressed at the whole family rather than the alcoholic individual alone. Thus, for example, the assessment phase of treatment would typically be carried out via conjoint interviews of the whole family and/or important subunits (especially the marital dyad) with an eye toward obtaining the multiple perspectives of all family members on the history of alcohol use and its impact on individuals and relationships within the family. Also included here was a thorough exploration of the pros and cons of alcohol use for the family as a whole. This ability to obtain multiple perspectives is especially valuable in assessing the effect of intoxicated behavior on family regulatory mechanisms (as discussed earlier, these mechanisms include family problem-solving styles, daily routines, and family rituals).

In that a key aspect of this family systems therapy approach posits that understanding differences between patterns of interactional behavior in the presence versus the absence of active drinking is critical to the ultimate success of treatment, obtaining this history from the entire

TABLE 1. A Family Systems Treatment Model for Alcoholism

Family Systems Treatment Model for Alcoholism

I. Assessment

- Patterns of drinking
- Family characteristics
- Substance use/Family "goodness of fit"
- Pros and Cons of substance use

II. Family-level Detoxification

III. Post-Detoxification Period

- Establishing a secure environment for change
- Anticipating "lapses and relapses"
- Reinstituting alcohol-free routines and rituals

IV. Family vs. Individual Recovery

- Integrated family and individual recovery
- Redefining family identity
- The role of recovery

family is vastly preferable to interviewing the alcoholic family member alone. The provocative concept here is that a failure to appreciate and understand the complex ways in which alcohol-related behaviors have become incorporated in family life may paradoxically lead to an inadvertent destabilization rather than improvement of family life following the removal of alcohol secondary to participation in an alcoholism treatment program.

The most radical component of the treatment model, however, was the concept of *family-level detoxification.* Simply put, the idea was that if the family was now in effect an alcoholic system (a behavioral system organized around alcohol use-abuse), then it was the whole family that needed to be detoxified. That is, the primary goal would be not only cessation of drinking on the part of the alcoholic patient, but the establishment of an alcohol-free family environment as well (see Table 2).

To accomplish this aim, a multiphase process was suggested, comprised of six integrated components: (1) the development of a written contract–the family detoxification contract–conjointly constructed by the family and the therapist; (2) the use of a core set of metaphors

TABLE 2. The Components of Family-Level Detoxification

Principles of Family-Level Detoxification

I. Therapist Stance

- Use of non-blaming, non-pathologizing language in exploring alcohol-related behaviors (pros and cons of alcohol use)
- Use of collaborative stance to facilitate joining with family against alcohol (externalization)

II. Goals

- Making the biological environment of the "identified patient" alcohol-free
- Making the psycho-social environment of the "identified patient" alcohol-free

III. Phases of Detoxification

- Physiological detox and home environment detox
- Extended family and social network

IV. Central Techniques

- The detoxification contract
- Making the contract public
- Rehearsing behavior in high-risk environments

around which the detoxification contract is framed; (3) a multistage strategy for implementing the scope of detoxification; (4) the use of public disclosure to reinforce the meaning and importance of the detoxification contract; (5) the use of a prospective, anticipatory stance to identify potential challenges to abstinence; and (6) ample rehearsal of strategies to effectively meet these potential challenges to abstinence.

Also important here was the suggested stance to be taken by the therapist in facilitating the creation of the family detoxification contract, a stance that emphasized two major components: (a) the use of non-blaming, non-pathologizing language in exploring the pros and cons of alcohol use and alcohol-related behaviors for both alcoholic and non-alcoholic family members; and (b) the use of a collaborative approach to facilitate joining with the family against on-going alcohol use (in other words, helping the family to differentiate between alcohol abuse and the alcohol abuser–what family therapists call *externalization* of the symptom).

By asking the couple to work together on framing the contract and by establishing as the treatment goal the metaphor of an alcohol-free family environment, the therapist is automatically reframing the entire alcoholism issue in family rather than individual terms. It is in this way that the family detoxification contract differs from other contracting approaches that have been used successfully by behavioral family therapists in treating substance abuse, for example, the versions of the Antabuse (disulfiram) contract advocated by a number of clinical researchers (Keane et al., 1984; O'Farrell & Bayog, 1986). Although the therapist is not disputing that the IP has been consuming the alcohol, he/she is dramatically reinforcing the concept that alcoholism has in important ways taken over family life. Thus, at the same time that this phase of treatment is aimed at the important goal of cessation of drinking (as a necessary prerequisite for further treatment), the therapist is also carrying out essential reframing work to enable the couple to reorganize family life so that the necessary relapse prevention tools and structures are in place.[2]

Family Belief Systems and Motivation Interviewing: In its original conceptualization, family-level detoxification had as its goal the *actual* removal of alcohol from the family system. Thus the contract that was negotiated with the family typically included abstinence on the part of the IP, making the family's home alcohol-free, and negotiating with all family members that they would not consume alcohol at family events (whether inside or outside the home). In other words, the dual goals of the detoxification contract–to make the biological environment of the IP and the social environment of the family alcohol-free–was interpreted literally in the discussions carried out with the family as part of determining how the detoxification contract was to be implemented.

Whereas in its initial conceptualization, our treatment model was primarily influenced by findings from empirical studies emphasizing those aspects of behavior thought to play a role in regulating (patterning) family life, as the model evolved the emphasis switched to a focus on *family belief systems*. Although we had for some time been describing the sober-intoxicated cycling in interactional states that we had observed in alcoholic families as a process that acted "as if" the family had come to believe that certain behaviors were only accessible if alcohol was present, we now began to directly engage the issue of the *actual* belief systems held by the family about alcohol use and its behavioral consequences.

Previously we were focused almost entirely on the interactional behaviors themselves; now we were looking at the belief systems *behind* these behaviors. And as a consequence, it was no longer sufficient to simply observe family behavior as part of the assessment process. We now had to also utilize techniques that allowed us to access family belief systems. It was at this juncture that the merger of our family systems assessment techniques with the approaches advocated by Miller, Rollnick and others as part of what they called Motivational Interviewing became so attractive (Miller & Rollnick, 2002). At the same time, the challenge was how to adapt the MI approach, which assumed a dyadic and dialectic process between interviewer and subject, to a setting in which the interviewer was hearing the perspectives (gathering data) from multiple sources (that is, more than one family member).

Influenced by this new challenge, our prior treatment approaches have undergone important alterations. For example, the concept of family-level detoxification, which had taken literally the goal of making the family environment alcohol-free, was now reconceptualized as focusing instead on "detoxifying" the family's *organization around alcohol*. Thus the target was the family's belief system that alcohol not only was a central organizing principle for behavior within the family, but also that this role for alcohol in family life was essentially non-negotiable. Within the new language we were now using with families, such a belief could be presented to the family as a "failure of imagination" on their part–that is, a rigid belief system that alcohol was a necessary ingredient in order for certain adaptive behaviors to be activated/accessed.

In other words, these family-level belief systems about the family's inability to function without alcohol could easily be seen as family-level versions of what the MI advocates were calling a person's doubts about his or her ability to change. But this time we are saying that it is the family, as well as the alcoholic individual, that is unable to imagine what life would look like without alcohol. It is this combination of the pessimism about the ability to affect the IP's drinking behavior, the belief that the family *needs* the behaviors activated during the intoxicated interactional state, and the inability to imagine any truly compelling alternative to alcohol as the central organizing principle in family life that creates the rigidity and chronicity of behavior the therapist engages when the family presents for treatment.

Combining Family Systems and MI Concepts: Central to the motivational-enhancement treatment approach is the emphasis on ambivalence about change (Miller et al., 1992). In the MET approach, ambivalence stems from two different sources–reluctance to give up what are thought of as positive aspects of substance use, and an underlying belief that change is not in fact possible (the belief that I simply can't do it, so why try).

A combined family systems/motivational interviewing approach adds an important additional element to this formula–its emphasis on the importance of an understanding of sober-intoxicated cycling as a fundamental behavior pattern existing at the family level. This emphasis is key to the model because central to our understanding of why families are often so ambivalent about tackling substance abuse change is a purported family-level belief system that behaviors only accessible in the presence of alcohol are essential to the family's ability to successfully manage key problems in their lives.

Thus the issue may not be so much "can I stop using"–a concept in the MET understanding of why people don't undertake behavior change–but rather, "if we change, we will no longer have the necessary resources to manage/solve/neutralize important problems in our lives." In other words, what is hypothesized to be core here is a *family belief system* about the extent to which alcohol is a necessary component of successful family problem-solving.

At a relatively simple level, we all ascribe to such belief systems about alcohol. "If I have a drink first, it will loosen me up and I'll be more relaxed and more companionable at the party." "If you want to see me at my funniest, just give me a beer or two." At some point, however, if a belief takes hold that one can *only* behave in a particular way if alcohol is present, and if the behavior itself is positively connoted, then at that point we are justified in saying that this person has incorporated a belief in alcohol as having important potential adaptive components for successful functioning.

The family systems model takes this concept an important step further. It proposes not only that such beliefs are present at a family level, but also that they are so central to behavior in a family organized around alcohol that the family behaves *as if* it believes that it can only access critical family-level interactional behaviors if alcohol is present. However, even if this belief system exists for the family, it may well be the case that the belief that it is only in the intoxicated interactional state that the family can access certain adaptive behaviors is open to challenge. That is, whether intoxication is a necessary component for short-term problem solving is exactly the type of belief that can be open for discussion in the same way motivational interviewing looks for examples of behaviors that might raise doubts in a person's mind about a belief that he or she is incapable of stopping or reducing alcohol use.

As explicated by Miller and Rollick, MI has five basic principles that underscore the approach to be taken by the therapist treating a patient with a substance abuse problem: (1) *express empathy* about the patient's condition; (2) *develop discrepancy* regarding the patient's beliefs about his/her behavior; (3) *avoid argumentation* with the patient about continued alcohol use; (4) *roll with the patient's resistance* to change; and (5) *support patient self-efficacy* regarding decisions about behavior change. It would be our contention that every one of these principles is compatible with a family therapy approach to alcoholism treatment. In fact, what is being described in the MI approach is the same type of collaborative, non-pathologizing therapeutic stance that was being advocated when we used the metaphor of the clinician-researcher to describe how a family systems therapist should interact with an alcoholic family.

THE SYSTEMIC-MOTIVATIONAL MODEL (SMM) OF TREATMENT

How then might a treatment model based on the combination of family systems and motivational enhancement principles be formulated? Our current version of a systemic motivational model of treatment envisions treatment proceeding through three distinct phases: (1) an Assessment/Consultation phase in which the main task is working with family members to examine their current views about alcohol use and abuse, and to ready the family for possible change; (2) a Family-Level

Treatment phase in which the family develops and implements an action plan centered around altering the ways in which alcohol is used and abused; and (3) an Aftercare and Relapse Prevention phase in which the family institutes alcohol-free routines and rituals, makes decisions about involvement with recovery/rehabilitation programs, and makes decisions about whether to reorganize around non-alcohol related family themes moving forward.

A brief description of the goals and strategies for each of these treatment phases follows. Note that each of the phases still draws heavily on concepts originally explicated in our Family Life History treatment model (Steinglass et al., 1987), but this time also incorporates important principles from the Motivational Enhancement Treatment model (Miller & Rollnick, 2002), especially the weight given to a thorough exploration of the pros and cons of continuing alcohol use (ambivalence about change), and the neutrality taken by the therapist about continued drinking (the incorporation of harm reduction as a viable treatment goal).

The Assessment/Consultation Phase: Once again, the assessment phase is carried out via a series of conjoint family interviews (including the alcoholic family member). During these interviews, the therapist starts with the usual review of issues that bring the family to treatment—issues that may or may not initially include alcohol abuse. The therapist positions him/herself as a consultant to the family, and early on focuses attention not only on family concerns, but also on family resources and examples of successful family management of prior problems. In this way, the collaborative, non-pathologizing stance that is a core feature of the SMM approach is rapidly established.

Assuming that the focus will then shift to concerns about alcohol use (usually described as the alcoholic family member's problem), the interviewing process instead reframes the "problem" as a family-level issue by questioning the family about its prior history vis-à-vis alcohol and exploration of the role of alcohol use in family life (with a particular focus on the relationship between alcohol use and the family regulatory behaviors of routine, rituals, and problem-solving strategies).

Emphasis is placed on family-level belief systems about alcohol and alcoholism, and on encouraging the family to explore the pros and cons *both* of continuing alcohol use *and* of eliminating alcohol use from family life. With all family members contributing ideas it is possible not only to generate a rich tableau of the role of alcohol use in family life, but also to help the family to see in what ways alcohol use has inserted itself in multiple aspects of family life. A corollary process that usually occurs is that the focus moves away from the alcoholic family member as the source of the problem, to a more nuanced and textured view of the ways in which all family members have a stake in both sides of the alcohol-present/ alcohol-absent dichotomy (that is, to help bring to the surface the ambivalence of all family members about change).

It is via this process that a secure environment for behavioral change (both individual and family-level) is established. Consonant with the principles of motivational interviewing, the therapist stays with an exploration of the pros and cons of change until it is clear to the family that the potential positive consequences of change significantly outweigh negative consequences, but also that the family's growing awareness of its internal and external resources and past history of successful problem solving help resolve its ambivalence about the possibilities of change vis-à-vis alcohol use.

Put in the terms of the Transtheoretical Model of Change (TTM), the therapist is utilizing the full power of family-level conversations to generate both multiple perspectives about the family's current situation and a multiplicity of ideas about potential strategies for change. It is hypothethized that this process not only facilitates more rapid movement from precontemplation→contemplation→preparation for action, but also helps support maintenance of change once it occurs because the "action plan" to follow has been generated by the whole family.

The Family-Level Treatment Phase: This phase parallels comparable phases in traditional treatment models in that its primary task is to generate and implement an action plan for change. Where it differs, of course, is that the action plan is both devised by the family as a group and then carried out utilizing all family members, ideally working in concert.

The default action plan would still be the family-level detoxification approach we originally developed as the core change component of the FLH treatment model. However, because many families are reluctant to embrace this approach as the first action step (usually because of the reluctance of non-alcoholic family members to implement the goal of establishing an alcohol-free family environment until less "drastic" options are first explored), in the SMM we are instead utilizing a version of a harm reduction approach in which the therapist takes on the educational role of reviewing for the family a menu of change options, and discusses the pros and cons of each with the family (that is, encourages the family to generate pro and con lists for each option).

An important component of these discussions is to encourage the family to identify a set of "outcome measures" that could be used to evaluate whether the particular action plan the family chooses is in fact working. The metaphor of the action plan as a research project is often a useful one here. The family and therapist are working as colleagues researching the potential effectiveness of the treatment action plan in achieving the outcome goals the family wants to accomplish. Anticipating possible problems in implementing the action plan would be part of these discussions, as would be how to enlist support from extended family and friendship networks in implementing the plan.

Once the plan has been drafted, therapy focuses on reviews of the family's progress in carrying it out. Critical here has been the ability of the therapist to reinforce the message that the plan belongs to the family, not the therapist. That is, it is the family that has devised the plan. Thus the therapist's role remains one of consultant to the family, assisting in evaluating how well the plan is working and how to continually improve it. In those instances where little progress is being made toward changing alcohol use, the therapist's job becomes one of supporting the family in returning to further "assessment" discussions, on the assumption that important data have yet to be uncovered (especially regarding family belief systems about alcohol use/abuse and its role in family life). This is the family-level version of staying at the appropriate stage of change in the TTM approach advocated by Miller and colleagues in the MET model.

The Aftercare and Relapse Prevention Phase: As with all relapse prevention approaches, the main goal of this phase of the systemic-motivational model is to maintain the changes that have occurred as a result of a successful action plan. Many treatment models have components designed to engage families as part of aftercare and relapse prevention. Some of the better known and researched are the spouse involvement approaches designed by McCrady and colleagues (McCrady et al., 1991; McCrady, Epstein, & Kahler, 2004), and the Counseling for Alcoholic Marriages (Project CALM) treatment protocol (O'Farrell, Choquette, & Cutter, 1998; Rotunda & O'Farrell, 1997).

At the same time, it is also the case that integrating traditional recovery approaches (especially 12-step programs) with family systems approaches has proven challenging. In part this is because traditional recovery programs typically establish separate tracks for alcoholic and non-alcoholic family members (e.g., AA and Al-Anon). In part it may be attributable to the hostility to the harm reduction approach expressed by many in the recovery community.

Nevertheless, it is clearly important that better bridges be built between family systems and traditional recovery approaches. Alcoholism, as is the case for all substance abuse disorders, is a chronic and often relapsing condition. Thus families coping with these conditions are "in for the long haul" and treatment, to be deemed successful, must be flexible enough to allow families room to balance their need for stability with their desire for developmental change, adaptability in the face of loss, etc.

We therefore approach the aftercare phase as one in which families not only have to evaluate the role of traditional recovery programs in their lives, but also have to carry on conversations about the extent to which they want to emphasize containment of the threat of alcohol abuse relapse versus emphasizing non-alcohol related issues in their lives. In the better of all possible worlds both would be possible. But more often decisions have to be made about how to allocate limited family resources (time and money being the most important ones here). How to handle family conflicts and the normal hassles of daily living without potentially disrupting the recovery process is another issue often brought up by families for discussion during this phase of treatment.

Assuming that "family-level detoxification" has been successfully negotiated (either literally or via a "detoxification" of family belief systems), then the family now finds itself in unfamiliar territory in that many of the family behavior patterns that were either used in the service of containing the negative effects of substance abuse or were incorporated as part of family problem solving strategies can now be challenged (that is, are no longer necessary). But new patterns are not necessarily yet in place, nor has the family engaged what an alcohol-free environment means for family priorities and future values.

Thus one can look on this phase of treatment as an opportunity for families to re-examine their lives toward the goal of deciding if they want to return to pre-existing family values and priorities, to build their lives around the new values coming from the traditional treatment programs they may be involved with (especially AA and Al-Anon), or to aim toward an integrated approach that combines the best of both world views. For most families, this phase is experienced as a blank slate and is often a time of confusion and distress. Thus the role of the therapist during this time is usually one of establishing a holding environment for the family, giving them time to experiment together and evaluate which paths they want to follow in support of aftercare and relapse prevention.

A CLOSING COMMENT

The treatment model I have described in this paper is clearly a work in progress. But the integration of family systems and motivational interviewing techniques has thus far proved entirely compatible. Further, motivation interviewing carried out with families rather than just individuals has in my view also substantially strengthened the quality of data available to the therapist attempting to assess the overall impact of chronic alcoholism on both alcoholic and non-alcoholic family members. It has also provided a vehicle for families to generate their own solutions to the challenges of chronic alcohol abuse by helping them identify and mobilize already present resources within the family.

Family therapists have long advocated what they call "both/and" solutions to conflicts, as opposed to "either/or" solutions. That is, the goal in a family therapy session is to generate ideas that encompass and take advantage of the multiple perspectives of all family members, rather than engage in discussions geared to choosing amongst ideas that are presented as if they are in competition with one another. In the alcoholism treatment arena, we often talk as if our ideas are of the second variety–competing approaches. But most treatment facilities use an eclectic approach in which a large menu of psychotherapies, pharmacotherapies, and adjunctive therapies are combined with 12-step approaches. At times these approaches are well integrated. But as often as not, they operate from different perspectives, utilizing different languages and values as well as different concepts about the causes of chronic alcoholism.

One of the steps forward offered by motivational interviewing is its suggestion that a common set of parameters can be identified separating successful from unsuccessful therapies. These parameters, Miller and colleagues have argued, have to do with therapist characteristics, centered around a non-confrontational, non-judgmental style that also focuses on therapist empathy (Miller, Benefield, & Tonigan, 1993). Because these are the very characteristics that have been emphasized in newer approaches to family therapy, family systems and motivation interviewing techniques would appear to be fully compatible and complimentary. And substance abuse disorders would appear to be an ideal set of conditions to use for testing out the potential power of this therapeutic marriage.

NOTES

1. The family systems model of alcoholism referred to here was first developed in conjunction with my colleagues Steven Wolin, Linda Bennett and David Reiss at the Center for Family Research, George Washington University School of Medicine, and subsequently refined in conjunction with my colleagues Sari Kutch and Gayna Havens at the Center for Substance Abuse and the Family of the Ackerman Institute for the Family.

2. A manualized version of a family systems treatment approach based in part on the model described above was, developed by Shoham and her colleagues (Rohrbaugh et al., 1995) in conjunction with the only controlled clinical trial to date of a family systems approach for alcoholism (Shoham et al., 1998).

REFERENCES

Baucom, D. H., Shoham, V. K. T., Mueser et al. (1998). Empirically supported couple and family interventions for marital distress and adult mental health problems. *Journal of Consulting and Clinical Psychology, 66,* no. 1:53-88.

Bennett, L. A., Wolin, S. J. Reiss, D. & M. A. Teitelbaum. (1987). Couples at risk for transmission of alcoholism: Protective influences. *Family Process,* 26:111-29.

Edwards, M. E., & P. Steinglass. (1995). Family therapy treatment outcomes for alcoholism. *Journal of Marital and Family Therapy,* 21, no. 4: 475-509.

Galanter, M. (1999). *Network Therapy for Alcohol and Drug Abuse.* New York: Guilford Press.

Garrett, J., J. Landau-Stanton, M. D. Stanton, J. Stellato-Kabat, & D. Stellato-Kabat. (1997). ARISE: A method for engaging reluctant alcohol- and drug-dependent individuals in treatment. *Journal of Substance Abuse Treatment,* 14, no. 3: 235-48.

Keane, T. M., D. W. Foy, B. Nunn, & R. G. Rychtarik. (1984). Spouse contracting to increase Antabuse compliance in alcoholic veterans. *Journal of Clinical Psychology,* 40: 340-44.

Landau, J., M. D. Stanton, D. Brinkman-Sull, D. Ikle, D. McCormick, J. Garrett, G. Baciewicz, R. R. Shea, A. Browning, and F. Wamboldt (2004). Outcomes with the ARISE approach to engaging reluctant drug and alcohol-dependent individuals in treatment. *American Journal of Drug and Alcohol Abuse,* 30, no. 4.

Lipps, A. J. (1999). Family therapy in the treatment of alcohol related problems: A review of behavioral family therapy, family systems and treatment matching research. *Alcoholism Treatment Quarterly,* 17, no. 3: 13-23.

Marlatt, G. A. (ed.). (1998). *Harm Reduction: Pragmatic Strategies for Managing High risk behaviors.* New York: Guilford Press.

Marlatt, G. A. and J. Gordon. (1985). *Relapse Prevention: Maintenance Strategies in the Treatment of Addictive Behaviors.* New York: Guilford Press.

Marlatt, G. A. & S. F. Tapert. (1993). Harm reduction: Reducing the risks of addictive behaviors. In *Addictive behaviors across the life span: Prevention, treatment and policy issues,* edited by A. Baer, G. A. Marlatt, and R.J. McMahon, 243-73. Newbury Park, CA: Sage.

McCrady, B. S., E. E. Epstein, & C. W. Kahler. (2004). Alcoholics Anonymous and relapse prevention as maintenance strategies after conjoint behavioral alcohol treatment for men: 18-month outcomes. *Journal of Consulting and Clinical Psychology*, 75, no. 5: 870-78.

McCrady, B. S., R. Stout, N. Noel, D. Abrams, and H. F. Nelson. (1991). Effectiveness of three types of spouse-involved behavioral alcoholism treatment. *Addiction*, 86, no. 11: 1115-24.

Meyers, R. J., W. R. Miller, D. E. Hill, & J. S. Tonigan. (1999). Community reinforcement and family training (CRAFT): Engaging unmotivated drug users in treatment. *Journal of Substance Abuse*, 10: 291-308.

Miller, W. R., R. G. Benefield, & J. S. Tonigan. (1993). Enhancing motivation for change in problem drinking: A controlled comparison of two therapist styles. *Journal of Consulting and Clinical Psychology*, 61, no. 3: 455-61.

Miller, W. R., R. J. Meyers, & J. S. Tonigan. (1999). Engaging the unmotivated in treatment for alcohol problems: A comparison of three strategies for intervention through family members. *Journal of Consulting and Clinical Psychology*, 67, no. 5: 688-97.

Miller, W. R. & S. Rollnick. (2002). *Motivational Interviewing, 2nd edition*. New York: Guilford Press.

Miller, W. R., A. Zweben, C. C. DiClemente, & R. G. Rychtarik. (1992). *Motivational Enhancement Therapy Manual: A clinical research guide for therapists treating individuals with alcohol abuse and dependence*. NIAAA Project MATCH Monograph Series Volume 2, vol. DHHS Publication No. (ADM) 92-1894. Rockville, MD: National Institute on Alcohol Abuse and Alcoholism.

O'Farrell T. J., K. A. Choquette, & H. S. G. Cutter. (1998). Couples relapse prevention sessions after behavioral marital therapy for male alcoholics: Outcomes during the three years after starting treatment. *Journal of Studies on Alcohol*, 59:357-370.

O'Farrell, T. J. & W. Fals-Stewart. (2002). Alcohol abuse. In *Effectiveness research in marriage and family therapy*, edited by D.H. Sprenkle, 123-61. Alexandria, VA: American Association for Marriage and Family Therapy.

O'Farrell, T. J. & R. D. Bayog. (1986). Antabuse contracts for married alcoholics and their spouses: A method to maintain Antabuse ingestion and decrease conflict about drinking, 1-8.

Reiss, D., R. Costell, H. Berkman, & C. Jones. (1980). How one family perceives another: The relationship between social constructions and problem-solving competance. *Family Process*, 19: 239-56.

Rohrbaugh, M. J., V. Shoham, C. Spungen, L. E. Beutler, & P. Steinglass. (1995). Family systems therapy in practice: A systemic couples therapy for problem drinking. In *Comprehensive textbook of psychotherapy: Theory and practice*, edited by B. Bongar and L.E. Beutler, 228-53. New York: Oxford University Press.

Rotunda, R. J., & T. J. O'Farrell. (1997). Marital and family therapy of alcohol use disorders: Bridging the gap between research and practice. *Professional Psychology: Research and Practice*, 28, no. 3: 246-52.

Rotunda, R. J., D. G. Scherer, & P. S. Imm. (1995). Family systems and alcohol misuse: Research and the effects of alcoholism on family functioning and effective family interventions. *Professional Psychology: Research and Practice*, 26, no. 1: 95-104.

Shoham, V., M. J. Rohrbaugh, T. R. Stickle, & T. Jacob. (1998). Demand-withdraw couple interaction moderates retention in cognitive-behavioral versus family-systems treatments for alcoholism. *Journal of Family Psychology*, 12, no. 4: 1-21.

Sisson, R. W., & N. H. Azrin. (1986). Family member involvement to initiate and promote treatment of problem drinkers. *Journal of Behavior Therapy and Experimental Psychiatry*, 17: 15–21.

Stanton, M. D., & A. W. Heath. (2005). Family/couples approaches to treatment engagement and therapy. In *Substance abuse: A comprehensive textbook, 4th edition*, edited by J. H. Lowinson, P. Ruiz, R. B. Millman, and J. G. Langrod, 680-90. Baltimore: Lippincott Williams & Wilkins.

Steinglass, P. (1979). The Home Observation Assessment Method (HOAM): Real-time naturalistic observation of families in their homes. *Family Process*, 18: 337-54.

—. (1980). A life history model of the alcoholic family. *Family Process*, 19: 211-25.

—. (1981). The alcoholic family at home: Patterns of interaction in dry, wet and transitional stages of alcoholism. *Archives of General Psychiatry*, 38: 578-84.

Steinglass, Peter, L. A. Bennett, S. J. Wolin, & D. Reiss. (1987). *The alcoholic family*. New York: Basic Books.

Steinglass, P., D. I. Davis, & D. Berenson. (1977). Observations of conjointly hospitalized "alcoholic couples" during sobriety and intoxications: Implications for theory and therapy. *Family Process*, 16: 1-16.

Thomas, C. and J. Corcoran. (2001). Empirically based marital and family interventions for alcohol abuse: A review. *Research on Social Work Practice*, 11, no. 5: 549-75.

Velleman, R. (2006). The importance of family members in helping problem drinkers achieve their chosen goal. *Addiction Research and Theory*, 14, no. 1: 73-85.

Wolin, S. J., L. A. Bennett, & D. L. Noonan et al. (1980). Disrupted family rituals: A factor in the intergenerational transmission of alcoholism. *Journal of Studies on Alcohol*, 41: 199-214.

doi:10.1300/J020v26n01_02

Beyond "Happily Ever After": Family Recovery from Alcohol Problems

Joyce Schmid, PhD, MFT
Stephanie Brown, PhD

SUMMARY. Based on the findings of the Family Recovery Project, stages and domains of family recovery from alcoholism are described, illustrated by an ongoing hypothetical family case example. The characteristics of each stage are presented, along with major principles of treatment for each stage. The stages of family recovery parallel the stages of individual recovery from alcoholism, and therapists use different approaches in each recovery stage. Families benefit from understanding the process of recovery and knowing what to expect in each stage. Recovery is traumatic as the alcoholic family system collapses. Outside supports, especially Twelve-Step programs, are essential to allow families to negotiate this trauma. The care of children is a special challenge as families go through recovery. doi:10.1300/J020v26n01_03 *[Article copies available for a fee from The Haworth Document Delivery Service: 1-800-HAWORTH. E-mail address: <docdelivery@haworthpress.com> Website: <http://www.HaworthPress.com> © 2008 by The Haworth Press. All rights reserved.]*

Joyce Schmid is a psychotherapist in private practice in Menlo Park, CA.
Stephanie Brown is Director of The Addictions Institute in Menlo Park, CA and Research Associate at the Mental Research Institute (MRI) in Palo Alto, CA.
Address correspondence to: Dr. Joyce Schmid, 830 Menlo Avenue, Menlo Park, CA 94025.

[Haworth co-indexing entry note]: "Beyond 'Happily Ever After': Family Recovery from Alcohol Problems." Schmid, Joyce, and Stephanie Brown. Co-published simultaneously in *Alcoholism Treatment Quarterly* (The Haworth Press) Vol. 26, No. 1/2, 2008, pp. 31-58; and: *Family Intervention in Substance Abuse: Current Best Practices* (ed: Oliver J. Morgan, and Cheryl H. Litzke) The Haworth Press, 2008, pp. 31-58. Single or multiple copies of this article are available for a fee from The Haworth Document Delivery Service [1-800-HAWORTH, 9:00 a.m.-5:00 p.m. (EST). E-mail address: docdelivery@haworthpress.com].

KEYWORDS. Alcohol, family, recovery, therapy

INTRODUCTION

In this chapter, which is based on the findings of the Family Recovery Project (Brown and Lewis, 1999), we describe the stages of family recovery from alcoholism. After a brief historical orientation to the field of family alcoholism treatment, we follow a recovering alcoholic family through drinking and the stages of recovery. For each stage, we describe the expectable environment, characteristics of the family system, the state of individual development, and finally, treatment considerations.

BRIEF HISTORICAL OVERVIEW
OF TREATMENT FOR THE ALCOHOLIC FAMILY

For years, alcoholism research and treatment focused only on the drinker, the alcoholic, and only on active drinking, alcoholism. There was widespread agreement that the goal of treatment should be abstinence and that abstinence would signal the end of the problem. But as Brown's research with alcoholics revealed (Brown, 1985), the cessation of drinking is only a landmark in a long process of recovery for the alcoholic. She found that this process consists of predictable stages, with recognizable characteristics, and specific treatment principles at each stage.

Similarly, for years there was no research on the family except, for example, on the now-discredited idea that wives caused the alcoholism of their husbands (Fox, 1956; Edwards et al., 1973; Jackson, 1954, 1962) or on the ways that wives could support the alcoholic in recovery. Family members were not viewed as needing treatment for themselves, nor was alcoholism viewed as a family disease (Jackson, 1962).

The birth of Al-Anon (1984), the 12-step program that followed from Alcoholics Anonymous (Alcoholics Anonymous, 1955), set the seeds for change. Research and treatment for actively addicted families followed (Steinglass et al., 1987). In addition, the 1980s and 90s saw a groundswell of interest in individuals affected by the drinking of others. The "Adult Children of Alcoholics" movement (Brown, 1988, 1991, 1995; Brown et al., 1989; Cermak, 1989; Black, 1981) and the "codependency" literature (Cermak, 1986; Shaef, 1986) brought this interest to the fore.

The question remained, however: what happens to the alcoholic family–and all of its members–after the drinking stops?

FAMILY RECOVERY PROJECT

Brown and Lewis (1999) conducted an in-depth exploratory research undertaking called "The Family Recovery Project" in order to address this question. They studied 52 alcoholic couples and families with lengths of recovery ranging from 79 days to 18 years. Each couple or family was assessed by the following tools: a three hour interview (Brown and Lewis, 1999, Appendix A) which was both audiotaped and videotaped; five tests of individual and family function; and a demographic questionnaire (results in Brown and Lewis, 1999, Appendix B). In addition, three couples with long-term sobriety participated in an ongoing couples group which met monthly for five years and provided information about the process of recovery over time. Finally, a MAPS (Maintaining Abstinence Programs) curriculum was piloted on a group of couples and families with over a year of abstinence.

Analysis of the research data revealed that the end of the drinking itself does not end the family's problems, but rather is only a signpost in a long process of recovery for the whole family, just as it is for the alcoholic. Individual family members and the family as a whole move through the same stages as the recovering alcoholic, and here too, there are definable tasks and treatment approaches for each stage. Conceptualizing the recovery of a whole family is, however, more complicated than focusing only on the individual.

There are the perspectives of the alcoholic and of each family member to consider, as well as the functioning of the family system (Steinglass et al., 1987; Bateson, 1971), which shapes and is shaped by the individual members. Finally, the environment also needs attention. It includes non-verbal factors such as mood, tone and atmosphere that also shape and are shaped by the individuals and the family system.

To describe the process of family recovery, Brown and Lewis (1999) outline each stage as well as three "domains" of experience within each stage: the environment, the system and the individuals within. Following the case of a family through the stages of active alcoholism and recovery, we review the domains and appropriate tasks of treatment for each family member in each stage. The "Chase Family" is a composite of many families whose identities have been disguised for confidentiality reasons.

STAGES AND DOMAINS OF RECOVERY

The Family in the Drinking Stage

> Mr. and Mrs. Chase are consulting a psychotherapist about Julie, their phobic seven year old. Julie's sister, Anne, 11, has never had problems like this. She gets straight A's and cooks dinner every night, which is helpful because Mrs. Chase suffers from migraines. Mr. Chase is working so hard at the office that he has developed ulcers. The couple loves to socialize, enjoys wine tasting, and has an extensive collection of fine wines. While they insist that all they want is Cognitive Behavioral Therapy for Julie's problems, they are willing to participate in an evaluation by the therapist.
>
> The therapist learns that Mr. and Mrs. Chase go out to parties three times a week, drinking wine with friends. They leave Julie with Anne. Mr. Chase has received a series of poor reviews at work, and he comes home and drinks "a few" cocktails and a bottle of wine each night while watching television to deal with the job and financial stress. Julie is a handful for Mrs. Chase, and they end up in screaming fights. Mr. Chase tries to ignore them, but eventually storms in and yells at both of them. Anne disappears into her room to do her homework. With so much tension in the home and parents frequently yelling, the children are ashamed to bring friends home. There is no set bedtime or evening routine for the children, and both of them stay up quite late. When the therapist asks Mr. Chase about his drinking, he insists angrily that Julie has the problem, not he.

This family is in the "Drinking" stage of the disease of alcoholism. They are "caught in the double bind of active alcoholism. They are dominated and organized by the realities of drinking, which everyone must deny and explain at the same time" (Brown & Lewis, p. 103). Alcohol affects each "domain" of family life: the environment, the system, and individual development.

The Environment. The Chase home is characterized by tension, anxiety and emotional pain. The children's needs are neglected. There is hostility between Julie and her mother, and there is alternate disengagement and hostility between her father and the rest of the family. The drinking is rationalized: Dad needs to drink because of job stress. No one acknowledges that alcohol is a problem. There is a sense of impending doom as both Mr. and Mrs. Chase avoid dealing with the likely loss of his job.

The System. This family revolves around drinking. It is the focus of social life, and is seen by Mr. Chase as the solution to problems. Family rituals (Wolin et al., 1979, 1980) such as birthdays, holidays, vacations, and "relaxation" are built around alcohol and the effects of drinking. The family system is characterized by rigid rules–don't talk about the drinking, don't get dad upset, take over for mom. Roles are rigid and hierarchies are reversed, as Anne takes on adult responsibilities. Important rituals such as entertainment, relaxation, holidays and vacations are structured around drinking (Steinglass et al., 1987; Wolin et al., 1980). Boundaries between the family and the outside sober world are impermeable; the family isolated. The alcoholic is dominant in the family, and everyone reacts to him, trying to keep him from yelling.

Individual Development. Each family member becomes dominated and controlled by the needs of the drinker and the alcoholic system. Mr. Chase denies that he has a problem with alcohol and explains his continued drinking as a solution to his stress. Mrs. Chase agrees, trying hard to please her husband because he has so much work stress, and because when he is not pleased he yells at her. Although she herself does not enjoy drinking, she attends the wine parties because Mr. Chase likes them. She subordinates her needs, preferences and views of reality to the dominance of her husband. Her headaches may be a somatic response to the realities of drinking and all its consequences that she cannot acknowledge. The children tiptoe around their father. Anne puts her school involvement, her friendships, and her own emotions on hold in her frantic attempt to keep the family functioning. Julie is the only one to express anxiety openly and she is pathologized for doing so.

This situation is typical of an alcoholic family in the Drinking stage. The environment is unsafe, in a state of both acute and chronic trauma (Brown, 1994; Herman, 1992; Krystal, 1978; Khan, 1963). The family system is organized around protecting its members from the effects of drinking, and also around maintaining the drinking. Each family member subordinates the self to the dictates of the drinking family system and the dominance of the alcoholic, while the individual's perceptions, beliefs, feelings and needs are suppressed. Individual development, organized by defense, is arrested or skewed towards pathology, as family members try to deal with the conditions imposed by drinking. Attachment of the children to their parents, and of the couple to one another, is based on acceptance of the drinking and the denial of it at the same time.

This double bind solidifies the dominance of defense. Language is defensive. Words are used not to transmit information, but to keep someone from exploding and to deny the realities of alcoholism in the family. Family members fear that any acknowledgment of the realities would threaten the cohesiveness of the family, which, in fact, is likely true.

Treatment in the Drinking Stage. A key treatment principle for family members in the Drinking Stage, including the alcoholic, is to help them shift their focus away from others and from the preservation of the unhealthy system, onto themselves and their own needs, experiences, perceptions, behaviors, and feelings. They each need to acknowledge the reality of alcoholism in the family, their own role in perpetuating it, and its effect on them. How is such acknowledgment to be achieved? This is largely a cognitive task, requiring direct challenge of what is called "alcoholic thinking." "Alcoholic thinking" includes the distorted logic and false premises that the family has relied on to preserve their denial of alcoholism. The Chases, for example, demonstrate alcoholic thinking in their beliefs that the only problem in the family is Julie's phobia, and that Dad's drinking is a reasonable way of coping with stress.

The therapist needs to juxtapose facts in new ways, and to question the family's ideas of cause and effect so that the alcoholism in the family can be recognized. In working with the Chases, the therapist gently suggests that maybe Dad's drinking actually causes his stress, rather than the other way around. If there is resistance, psychodynamic techniques can be used to resolve roadblocks to knowing the reality of familial alcoholism. What conscious and unconscious factors contribute to everyone's defenses against knowing? What would happen if family members recognized the alcoholism and what would it mean to them for a family member to be alcoholic?

While the development of new cognitions would begin to destabilize the alcoholic system, and thereby open the road to recovery, the powerful forces of loyalty, attachment, and homeostasis fight against this knowledge. Protection of the alcoholic family system, which is experienced by family members as crucial to the survival of the family, requires the sacrifice of self, that is, of one's own abilities both to see the reality of alcoholism and to recognize the feelings engendered by it.

Consequently, for recovery to occur, the alcoholic family system must destabilize significantly and even collapse. The pathological sacrifice of the self to the dictates of the system must stop. But getting to a stopping point is difficult. As soon as the system is challenged, family members reflexively tighten their defenses. The isolated alcoholic family feeds on itself, reinforcing addictive behavior and the thinking that supports it. So individuals must reach outside of the family for the support and new perspectives necessary for recovery. Many kinds of outsiders– friends, coworkers, clergy and therapists–can offer outside influence. If an alcoholic family turns to a therapist, they are likely to ask for help with all the real problems that accompany drinking such as anxiety, depression and stress. The therapist, however, focuses on the drinking itself, and links it to the other problems. The therapist sees and talks about the realities that are denied. This must be done without blame and with a fair amount of tact.

It is our view that most therapeutic interventions at this stage should target the individuals, encouraging both self-focus and cognitive change. This type of intervention is necessary in order to reverse the sacrifices of self and of independent perception that characterizes and sustains the alcoholic family system. Family members, effectively muzzled within the family, may look to the therapist to see if permission is granted to see and know the truth. The therapist provides support for someone to step out of the family collusion and tell the truth as he sees it, so that the process of change can begin for everyone. This twin focus on the self and on drinking starts to erode denial that problem drinking is occurring. As drinking becomes a topic of conversation, the consequences of the drinking also become fair game. People's feelings begin to emerge. This principle of focusing on individual perceptions and feelings and on drinking and its consequences applies to treating the family as a whole or any subgroup or individual in the family.

As the realities of drinking are addressed, first the effects that feel positive to the drinker and the family, then gradually, the negatives as well, beliefs about cause and effect can be reversed. For example, "Mr. Chase, you said that you drink when you come home from work because you are tense. Have you ever thought that the tension could actually be the effect of your body withdrawing from the drinks you had yesterday?" Or, "Julie, you said your mother yells at you because you're bad. Maybe you feel you're bad because you're being yelled at." Or, "Mrs. Chase, you mentioned that it bothers you when Mr. Chase withdraws, and you said he withdraws when he's drinking. Why do you serve him drinks?"

While alcoholism is a brain disease (Nixon, 2006; Volkow and Li, 2005) that develops a life of its own in the body, there are also important psychological and social factors that both start and maintain alcoholic drinking. Investigation of these factors, utilizing a psychodynamic approach to understand conscious and unconscious conflict and past trauma, can help the alcoholic and family members gain insight into the realities of the drinking. Brown illustrates this kind of therapeutic intervention in a teaching film (Jaylen Productions, 1997). In this film, an alcoholic remembers the pain and anger he felt when his father drank. The experience of remembering both the images and the feelings of his childhood helps him to realize how his own drinking is affecting his children. In that crisis of connecting his past with his present, he recognizes that he has lost control, just like his father, and he moves into recovery.

Turning back to a cognitive approach, it is important to find out what the alcoholic or family members define as "alcoholism." Many people equate alcoholism with end-stage chronic drunkenness and assure themselves that they or their loved ones could not be alcoholic because they are not living under bridges. The therapist helps people see that their definition bolsters their denial and distortions. The therapist then educates them about the realities of the progression of the disease, accenting early signs and symptoms.

The needed collapse of the alcoholic family system can occur as a result of psychotherapy, as the rules and beliefs of the alcoholic system erode, and individuals change their behavior. For example, if Mrs. Chase were to learn to assert herself in the family, or maybe even to decide to leave, the family would function differently. Destabilization of the alcoholic system also can be triggered by the progression of the alcoholism itself. For example, if Mr. Chase were to lose his job, or if he were to get a citation for driving under the influence of alcohol (a "DUI"), or to hurt himself or someone else while driving, or if the neglect of the children were to become more extreme and come to the attention of the authorities, things would change and denial could be broken.

However it occurs, the collapse of the family system is a traumatic change. During the collapse and for a time afterwards, things are likely to get worse for the family, not better. But it is important that the therapist try to foment this change, and tolerate it when it occurs, rather than trying to restore the previous unhealthy equilibrium. The process of this collapse of the family system is called the "Transition" Stage.

The Family in the Transition Stage

The Transition Stage marks the family's shift from drinking to abstinence. In the first part of this stage–Drinking Transition–alcoholic thinking starts to change although the drinking continues. The drinker and/or family members begin to recognize and acknowledge their own loss of control, and that of others in the family. In the second part of Transition–Abstinent Transition–behaviors change. The alcoholic stops using alcohol, and/or family members adopt new ideas and behaviors vis-a-vis the drinking. This is nothing less than a revolution. And like any revolution, it is a time characterized by chaos, confusion, and lack of safety.

The old rules no longer apply, but there are not yet new ones. Even after the drinking has stopped, the family must continue to deal with its consequences, often in a more intensive way than had been necessary during the drinking. This can be extremely disappointing and discouraging for alcoholics and family members alike who often have believed that if the drinking would cease, they would live happily ever after. Instead, that family finds itself faced with the "trauma of recovery" (Brown and Lewis, 1999, p. 181).

Imagine a double arrow between the Drinking and Abstinent sub-phases of Transition as alcoholics and their families move from Abstinence back to Drinking and then back again to Abstinence. They recognize loss of control and enter Abstinence, then deny it once more in the face of overwhelming difficulty and pain without adequate supports, and return to Drinking. They return to Abstinence when they are forced again by negative consequences to face loss of control.

To envision the complexity of recovery for an alcoholic family, now consider that the alcoholic and each family member has his or her own trajectory in the process. This separate path of individual recovery will challenge family attachments that are built on maintaining pathology.

Drinking Transition

Julie Chase is referred for CBT, as requested by her family, and Mr. and Mrs. Chase decide to have couples therapy to help them parent Julie, who is now refusing to go to school. Mrs. Chase believes that Julie's therapy is making her worse and pulls her out. Mrs. Chase's headaches are becoming worse and more frequent, and the fights between her and Julie are intensifying. Mr. and Mrs. Chase are fighting more too, as disagreements about how to handle Julie's school refusal lead to screaming matches. Mr. Chase is warned that if his performance does not improve at work he will lose his job, and he increases his drinking to deal with the job stress.

He is referred by HR to a counselor who strongly confronts his drinking, and he drops out of counseling. One night on the way home from a party, Mr. Chase is stopped by the police for erratic driving, and is charged with a "DUI." He loses his license temporarily, is required to pay a fine, and is assigned to alcohol education groups and roadside cleanup. Although he is still drinking heavily, the alcohol education is having an effect, and he now secretly suspects that he is an alcoholic. He tells himself he could not be an alcoholic like his father, however; he has never hit anyone and he does not drink at bars as his father had done. After the DUI, Mrs. Chase continues to go to parties with him, but now she drives, and since she is driving, she does not drink. In order to drive Mr. Chase to work and back, she stops doing the family's laundry, and Anne picks up that job too. Anne is starting to get headaches.

Things are changing for the Chase family. Let's examine their situation now, domain by domain.

Environment. The pressure on this family is building. The consequences of the drinking are becoming harder to avoid: the DUI, the threat of job loss, Julie's behavior problems and Mrs. Chase's and Anne's headaches. There is more fighting, more disruption, more anxiety, more demands on everyone. Things are getting worse.

System. While the alcoholic system is mainly the same as it was during Drinking, we do see a few signs of change. While the alcoholic is still drinking, and is still the dominant member of the family, there is some challenge to his position as Mrs. Chase is now willing to stand up to him about dealing with Julie. Anne continues her parental role, with more work than is appropriate for a child. She is now making an indirect bid for attention and relief (her headaches). Mrs. Chase continues to attend drinking parties with her husband but she no longer drinks with him, which is a big change. The most important change is the family's new involvement with outside influences: a therapist and the legal system have entered their lives. As in the Drinking Stage, the needs of the children continue to be placed below the alcoholic's need to drink, and below the cohesion of the family unit.

Individual Development. Mr. Chase is starting to question his drinking as he suffers the consequences of his DUI and is being exposed to alcoholism education. He is wondering whether he may be an alcoholic, but he tries to dismiss the idea. Now that she is abstinent herself, Mrs. Chase is able to realize the extent of the drunkenness at the parties she and her husband attend. She is starting to realize that Mr. Chase's drinking has been a problem, but balks at actually acknowledging that he is an alcoholic. When Al-Anon is recommended to her, she insists that her husband has the problem, not she. Julie is signaling more loudly that something is terribly wrong as she refuses to go to school. Anne continues to throw herself into the breach to keep the family functioning, but her body is starting to cry for help. Despite these signs of incipient change, individual development, needs and feelings continue to be sacrificed to the alcoholic family system.

The experience of the Chase family is common to alcoholic families in the Drinking Transition stage. In this stage we see some signs of progress toward recovery in the thinking of family members: people start to question the drinking or their participation in aiding and abetting it. But the environment, the system and individual development are as badly off as they were during Drinking–and worse.

Treatment in the Drinking Transition Stage. Family members in the Drinking Transition Stage, as in the Drinking Stage, continue to need cognitive work: the linkage of drinking behaviors and thinking patterns with their consequences, and a shift in attention from others to the self. As people become aware of the drinking and its effects, and want to stop, the therapist switches focus, helping patients to adopt new behaviors that foster and support abstinence. Here too, as in the Drinking stage, blocks to changing cognitions or behaviors are resolved through psychodynamic methods. In doing this work, it is essential that the therapist have a long-term view of alcoholism recovery. The participants in the Brown and Lewis study report repeatedly that the worsening of the family's life was an integral part of their path to recovery (Brown & Lewis, 1999, Chapter 9). The therapist needs to know that it is normal for things to get worse, often much worse, before they get better. This knowledge helps the therapist to communicate hope, even nonverbally, to the patient(s), and to tolerate the family members' distress–and her own.

In Transition, someone in the family begins to link the drinking with its consequences, and to recognize loss of control. The alcoholic begins to see his loss of control over alcohol, and/or a family member starts to realize that she cannot control the alcoholic. The therapist encourages this process, and continues to help each individual link cause and effect. Timing of these interventions is crucial. As Brown and Lewis point out, "The therapist must always be careful not to go so fast that the patient intensifies her defenses, nor to go so slowly as to convey to the patient a lack of urgency in dealing with the seriousness and centrality of alcohol in her life" (Brown & Lewis, 1999, p. 182).

The recognition of loss of control is usually accompanied by guilt, shame, regret, sadness, fear, anxiety, and other painful feelings. The therapist needs to resist the temptation to try to comfort the patient by excusing or rationalizing the out of control behaviors, or by playing down the consequences of those behaviors. These painful feelings are normal accompaniments to the awareness of loss of control, and can motivate people to behave differently. Yet these feelings can also block or interrupt movement into recovery. If difficult feelings turn into major depression or immobilizing anxiety, direct treatment for these conditions may be necessary.

While it is crucial that the truth be faced by both patient and therapist, it is also essential that the patient's honesty be met by the therapist's acceptance, compassion and lack of judgment, and that the patient receive help in learning these stances toward himself as well. For example, as Mrs. Chase comes to understand the ways in which she has tolerated and even aided and abetted Mr. Chase's drinking, and the ways she has lost control herself and neglected her children, she will likely be devastated. The therapist's job is to help her remain aware of what she has done, while turning her towards help and recovery, instead of against herself. Education about the disease concept of addiction (Jellinek, 1960) is helpful in this effort. The therapist reminds all family members that they have been out of control as a result of having or coping with the disease of alcoholism, which affects the entire family. They have been doing their best to survive with the disease, but their methods have been counterproductive. They need to learn new behaviors and new thinking, with self-focus high on the list.

But focusing on the self is extremely difficult for members of an alcoholic family; they have all been taught that doing so is selfish, disloyal and dangerous. Their most basic attachments to the family as a whole and to one another are rooted in the abandonment of self. The therapist guides family members to people outside of the family for support in the radical change to self focus, and to learn a new understanding of reality and new behaviors to match the new truths. As denial erodes, family members can be encouraged to explore programs such as AA, Al-Anon, Ala-Teen, and Ala-Kid. Members of these organizations have lived through and are continuing to live through their own experiences of drinking and recovery. They mentor, teach, and model recovery, provide an outside perspective, and are available to form strong emotional bonds with newly recovering people.

Perhaps one of the greatest challenges to families in both active drinking and recovery is attending to the needs of the children. Their needs were not met during drinking, and now things may be worse. The therapist is alert to the need for structural support for the family. Are babysitters, tutors, housecleaners, cooks, or drivers needed? Can extended family, friends, or agencies provide assistance? While seeking help to provide safety and nurturance for the children, however, a therapist also needs to weigh the danger of shoring up the alcoholic family system and protecting the drinking.

Abstinent Transition

Mr. and Mrs. Chase come to couples therapy utterly distraught. Mrs. Chase opens by describing the crisis of the night before. Julie staged a tantrum, screaming that she would not go to school the next day. Mrs. Chase was yelling back at her. Mr. Chase, who had been drinking in the living room, raced up the stairs two at a time, kicked open the door, raged at Mrs. Chase, and pushed her onto the floor. This was the first instance of violence in the family. Anne, terrified, called the police. By the time they arrived, things had calmed down and they left without making an arrest. After they were gone, Mr. Chase stormed out of the house. Mrs. Chase went into her room and cried for several hours. Julie and Anne huddled together and fell asleep in Julie's bed.

In the therapy session, Mr. Chase is furious that Anne called the police. Gradually, though, he acknowledges that he had been out of control. The therapist gently points out that he has crossed the line into his own definition of alcoholism by knocking down Mrs. Chase. Mr. Chase's anger disappears, and he seems to crumple as he admits that after he left the house, he went to a bar. He sees that he is an alcoholic and needs to stop drinking. He has learned about AA at his alcoholism education class, and says that he plans to attend an AA meeting that night. Mrs. Chase insists and tearfully tells him that he can't go to AA meetings because she needs him at home in the evenings. When asked by the therapist how she feels about Mr. Chase's acknowledgment that he is an alcoholic, and his decision to stop drinking, she becomes angry at the therapist.

"You think my husband is an alcoholic and you want him to tell everybody!" When asked what it would mean if her husband were an alcoholic, and if other people knew, Mrs. Chase shoots back, "Well, he's not!" The therapist offers Mrs. Chase a referral for individual therapy where she can explore these feelings and begin to understand her need for her husband not to be an alcoholic.

Mr. Chase attends an AA meeting once a week for a month. He says he has no desire for alcohol. He tells his family he has will power, and can stay sober if he wants to. He assures Mrs. Chase that, in fact, he is not an alcoholic, because alcoholics do not have will power the way he does. He is now abstinent when he watches television in the evening. Mrs. Chase continues to complain about his evening AA meeting, saying she can't handle the family alone. Mr. and Mrs. Chase continue to attend their parties, although she continues to drive, and neither one is drinking. Julie is missing school, and fighting with Mrs. Chase about it, until Mrs. Chase takes to her room with her headaches. Anne too is now missing school because her headaches are worse. The next month, Mr. Chase receives notice that he has been laid off from his job.

The drinking has stopped and Mr. Chase has begun to attend AA. This is a positive development–but things are still getting worse.

Environment. Although Mr. Chase is no longer drinking, nothing has improved for this family. It is still characterized by lack of safety, discord, and neglect of the children. Mr. Chase's job loss increases the family anxiety, and the specter of financial disaster enters the picture.

The System. The family continues to revolve around Mr. Chase as Mrs. Chase and the girls worry that he will start drinking again. The rigid boundaries around the family are continuing to fray, as Mr. Chase adds AA to his outside influences. Alcohol is no longer a part of family rituals and the rituals themselves are in flux. How will the family celebrate birthdays without alcohol? What do you do on Christmas Day if you don't have eggnog? How do you say "Happy New Year" without champagne? Anne continues to assume parental duties as the adults avoid them. The children's emotional needs and many of their physical needs continue to be neglected, and both of them are silently crying out for help. The system is disorganized and in turmoil.

Individual Development. Mr. Chase's AA attendance is a step in the direction of his individual development. While he does see that drinking has been a problem for him, and he is currently not drinking, he still does not understand the loss of control that characterizes the disease of alcoholism, and he does not grasp his own loss of control. His attachment to a wife who insists that he is not an alcoholic makes it harder for him to hold on to that fact and to attend AA. While Mrs. Chase is now able to acknowledge that drinking is a problem in the family, and is no longer drinking herself, she refuses to believe that Mr. Chase has lost control and is an alcoholic. She wants him to drink "normally." She continues to defer to him and try to please him, and then rages that his drinking has ruined the family. She is not able to look at herself and her own loss of control. She needs individual work to safely explore her resistance to acknowledging her husband's loss of control and her own. Mrs. Chase does not want her husband to be an alcoholic. Why?

The children are still struggling without support or guidance, and are dodging their parents' explosiveness.

Treatment in the Abstinent Transition Stage. Even when the drinking stops, the alcoholic and the alcoholic family often need continued cognitive and psychodynamic work to help them acknowledge their loss of control. *Only when the cognitive shift has been made from a belief in control to an acceptance of loss of control will people be motivated to undertake the behavioral changes that support recovery.* This shift, called "surrender" (Brown, 1985, p. 116-117; Tiebout, 1944, 1953) will allow the therapy to move to a behavioral plane, as the alcoholic asks, "What do I do?" (Jaylen Productions, 1997). In Abstinent Transition, the individuals in the alcoholic family may move back and forth between surrender and a restored belief in control and the therapy shifts accordingly. Mr. Chase has not reached the point of surrender. The therapist uses a cognitive approach to help him recognize his loss of control, and also a psychodynamic stance to help him explore his resistance to recognizing it. What conscious and unconscious factors are in the way? Mrs. Chase also needs cognitive and dynamic work to help her tolerate recognition of Mr. Chase's loss of control, and her own. In addition, she needs to understand that she is desperate to pull Mr. Chase back into the old way of being, for fear of the unknown, even though she recognizes the negative effects of his drinking.

The Brown and Lewis study reveals that for alcoholic families, recovery is a strange and frightening terrain. The experiences of the families who participated in the study have generated a map of this terrain, which is contained in *The Family Recovery Guide: A Map for Healthy Growth* (Brown, Lewis, & Liotta, 2000). The book outlines the stages of alcoholism recovery, with personal examples and exercises that help individuals understand what is normal and expected in recovery and also helps them challenge their own continuing defenses. Identification with the experiences of others in the Drinking and Transition Stages, whether in meetings or through a book, validates the family's current experience of disruption and chaos. This reduces shame. Learning of the experiences of others in recovery shows the family the light at the end of the tunnel. This reduces anxiety and instills hope. A map of recovery can be helpful to Mr. and Mrs. Chase when their denial and resistance to surrender are weakening.

Because Mr. and Mrs. Chase need to be encouraged to focus on themselves, as a direct intervention into the alcoholic family system, it is a good time for both to see individual therapists familiar with active addiction and recovery. In couples work, the focus needs to be on alcohol and each person's relationship to alcohol and to the family system that is organized around maintaining alcoholic pathology. If the therapy were to be derailed onto the couple's relationship separate from the issue of alcohol, then the alcoholic system, built on avoiding the alcoholism and defensively focusing only on the secondary problems created by drinking would be strengthened.

Over the course of a normal couple relationship, the partners tend to move from the unbounded symbiosis typical of falling in love to a more differentiated stance towards one another. The wonderful feeling of "being one" with the other normally gives way to both acknowledgment of and need for difference. This movement is called "individuation" (Bader & Pearson, 1988). When a couple gets stuck in a symbiotic bond, the sacrifice of their individual needs, thinking, and actions for the sake of the relationship–the complete trumping of the "I" by the "we"–forestalls growth. Alternatively, if one member is ready to individuate and the other is not, problems ensue between them. For the alcoholic couple, symbiosis develops around alcoholism, a symbiosis that both requires and fosters drinking. If one partner starts to head toward recovery, the other can be expected to try to pull the recovering partner back into the alcoholic symbiosis, despite the suffering that has been created by the drinking. The therapist needs to break this symbiosis by encouraging each member of the couple to think independently about the drinking, and to act independently in terms of self-care. Such cognitive and behavioral freedom will strain and sometimes can break the couple's bond. This can be difficult for the therapist, especially a therapist seduced by the counter-transference that it is the therapist's job to keep the couple together.

It is not uncommon for couples to separate physically once either or both partners have broken denial of the alcoholism and of the loss of control. The separation can be temporary, with couples reuniting as their separate selves are strengthened in recovery, or permanent if one member stays in denial, or if too much damage has been inflicted during the drinking. Paradoxically, a therapist who is willing to help the partners separate emotionally and who is willing to tolerate their risk of separation can help provide the couple's best chance of staying together, if they are taught to reach for outside support such as that offered in Twelve-Step programs. These programs can provide a holding environment for the relationship as the partners grow individually.

To the extent that patients are able to recognize their own loss of control, 12-Step programs such as AA and Al-Anon can be extremely useful in helping them adopt new behaviors and thinking, and these programs support individuation. But the couple will often resist attending. While these programs are a powerful antidote to the shame, anxiety and isolation that torment the couple as alcoholism is identified, that very shame, anxiety and isolation also keep people from seeking help.

When an alcoholic or "codependent" (family member or friend of an alcoholic) sees her own loss of control and wants to change her behavior, but is unwilling to attend AA or Al-Anon, psychodynamic work can be helpful to explore the resistance. Perhaps the individual has conflicts about accepting the identity of alcoholic or co-alcoholic (or codependent), or is anxious and conflicted about the meaning of attending a 12-step group. Understanding what is feeding resistance to attendance can free people to try it out. For example, Mrs. Chase's resistance to Al-Anon was based on her fear of being weak or needy. Her parents had responded coldly to her expressions of emotion or pain, and had made it known that such displays disgusted them. She had an entrenched conviction that she was lovable only when she was handling things by herself, a conviction that her therapist repeatedly challenged. Mrs. Chase came to realize that she did not want to see herself or her husband as weak, which is exactly how she would see him if he were to accept his loss of control, identify as an alcoholic and go to AA. The same applied to her. If she accepted her loss of control over both him and herself, identified as a co-alcoholic and went to Al-Anon, she would see herself as weak and thus deserving of the contempt she remembers feeling from her parents.

The Family in Early Recovery

When an alcoholic or family member can maintain a stance of surrender, accept the identity as an alcoholic or co-alcoholic ("codependent"), and is able reliably to behave in ways that support healthy growth, including abstinence, Early Recovery for the individual is in place. When everyone in the family has reached this point, the entire family is in Early Recovery. Each individual is focused on the self, learning new abstinent behaviors and beliefs, and each is able to tolerate separation from others in the family in order to keep the focus on themselves.

The adults are also able to pay attention to their children as they get support to combine a focus on individual recovery with parenting responsibilities.

When some family members are in recovery and others are not, it may be hard to tell if this is a recovering family. If it is, the system is now dominated and organized by recovery rather than drinking. In Early Recovery, although the family system remains a vacuum, or disorganized and fragmented because the drinking structure has collapsed, the individuals are recovery-focused. Family members can tolerate the vacuum in the system and in their relationships. A family is in recovery when recovery itself has replaced alcohol as the central organizing principle of the family system (Brown & Lewis, 1999, p. 64), even if not everyone is in recovery and chaos may still reign.

> The Chases experienced seven months of abstinence, with Mr. Chase attending weekly AA meetings over his wife's objections. This created a feeling of distance between them, as Mr. Chase began to learn a language that was foreign to his wife, and to have a body of experience from which she was excluded.
>
> Then Mrs. Chase impulsively handed her husband a glass of wine at a party. Yes, she knew his drinking had been a problem, but he really was more fun after a few drinks, and she missed that. Without a blink, Mr. Chase drank the wine and kept on drinking. Mrs. Chase longed to feel close to her husband again, so she drank with him. They left the party drunk, and Mrs. Chase drove home, crashing into a tree and denting the car. Shaken, they continued on home, where they had a screaming fight which woke up the children.
>
> The next day Mr. Chase went to two AA meetings, spoke in each one, and listened in a new way. For the first time, he realized what his loss of control meant. He really was an alcoholic! Mr. Chase attended AA every day for several months as he immersed himself in new learning that he hadn't been able to absorb before even though he'd been abstinent. He began to stay after each meeting to socialize and go for coffee, as he had been advised to do by the therapist. He chose a sponsor—an AA member with experience of the program who could mentor him and help him "work" the twelve steps—and began meeting weekly with him.
>
> Mrs. Chase was aghast to realize that she had actually handed her husband a drink and driven the car while intoxicated herself. She had earlier accepted a referral for individual therapy, and had been working on the meaning to her of loss of control and of

alcoholism. Now, when her therapist suggested that she go to Al-Anon, she went, and found the meetings so helpful that she too began to attend one each day, and also began staying afterwards to talk and go for coffee. She and Mr. Chase stopped needing to go to parties with drinking friends as they made new friends in AA and Al-Anon.

At home, they strengthened their adult positions. They followed advice from their therapist and friends in the 12-Step programs about establishing parental authority that had long been missing. For example, they insisted that Julie attend school no matter how much she protested. When she left school early, or refused to attend, they withdrew privileges such as television, computer use, and allowance. If Julie tried to provoke her mother into a fight, her father supported her mother. When Julie escalated by threatening suicide, they made arrangements to send her to residential treatment which included a school curriculum. This proved unnecessary. Julie's suicide threats abated and her school attendance began to improve as she sensed her parents' new connection, strength, and agreement on what they expected of her. She no longer felt as desperate to stay home and hold the family together. Mr. and Mrs. Chase arranged for her to attend a therapy group for children of alcoholics.

In addition, Mr. and Mrs. Chase began to structure regular homework time and bedtime for Anne, as they relieved her of her household duties. Mrs. Chase began to make dinner herself or to bring it home. The family began to eat together at an earlier hour so a parent could go to a meeting. Family members now shared household chores. Both of the children were now more protected and more able to focus on their own age-appropriate development. But everything was not rosy for the family. They were worried about finances since they had depleted their savings during Mr. Chase's unemployment. Julie still missed school at times and Anne was discovered drinking wine in her room.

Are these parents in Early Recovery? Now, at last, they are. Their most recent experience of drinking after a period of abstinence has graphically demonstrated to them their own loss of control, and has tipped them into the Early Recovery stage. In their fear of drinking again, they finally have embraced their identities as alcoholic and codependent, and have become willing to turn to something outside of themselves–in this case, their 12-Step programs–to keep them sober.

They have surrendered to the reality of alcoholism in the family and are taking behavioral steps to support sobriety. These are the hallmarks of Early Recovery. Let's look at the family in each domain.

The Environment. Mr. and Mrs. Chase are engaged in recovery activities, and they spend less time together. They are less volatile, so there is a much greater sense of calm in the home. But they also feel emotionally distant, something they'd been told to expect as they shifted their focus from each other onto themselves. They tolerate this sense of loss with the help of their recovery programs because they now understand the dangers of reconnection through drinking. The environment in Recovery is more "normal," but ironically, the new calm may stir up fears that were covered by all the chaos and the twin traumas of both active addiction and new abstinence–fear of both isolation and intimacy, fear of their own emotions, fear of relapse, fear for the future.

After their break in abstinence, the Chases have renewed their focus on active recovery. But the children are stressed by the chaos of increased recovery activities, as mom and dad center their lives around meetings and time with sponsors and recovering friends.

The System. In their new recoveries, life still revolves around alcohol– but now on *not* drinking. The Chases have shifted from familial isolation to acceptance of crucial support, leaving a vacuum within the home. The system continues in a state of collapse, though new structures based on recovery are beginning to take hold. The parents' assumption of responsibility has dramatically added containment where chaos had prevailed. The children are given schedules and rules, and are encouraged to relinquish their parental roles. In Early Recovery, families struggle to refrain from old ways of coping as new ways develop slowly.

Individual Development. Mr. and Mrs. Chase are deeply involved in their own recoveries. They are focusing on their own behaviors, feelings, needs. Now that they have fully accepted their loss of control, they are strengthening their individual recoveries and are less likely than they were before to sacrifice themselves by a return to the old system. When Mr. Chase feels the need to drink, he calls his sponsor or a recovering friend, takes a walk, or attends a meeting. Mrs. Chase is beginning to see that she does not have to be invulnerable and in control to be lovable. She realizes that she is a person in her own right and also that she is at least partially responsible for the family's problems. When she finds herself worrying that her husband will drink again, and blaming him, or when she is overcome with anxiety, she pulls out an Al-Anon reading to center herself, or calls her sponsor.

The children feel quite mixed about recovery. They were used to the independence that accompanies neglect and they miss it. At the same time, they still have to cope with often being left on their own. Anne, now almost 13, suffers from the loss of her important role as housekeeper. While her headaches have stopped, she is trying to deal with her despair by drinking. Julie is generally feeling better. Her attention and school work are both improving. No longer mother's scapegoat, she is much less anxious, but she sometimes feels empty and despondent. She tells her therapy group that she misses fighting with her mother.

Treatment in Early Recovery. At this stage, new behaviors of abstinence are firmly in place as are beliefs about loss of control and alcoholism. The therapist continues to monitor recovery programs, checking in on meetings and sponsorship, and addressing any problems in these areas. The main thrust of treatment continues to be behavioral and cognitive as individuals strengthen their healthy self-development. The therapist listens for a weakening or loss of the new identity as an alcoholic or a codependent. If pre-recovery misconceptions ("I am not an alcoholic, I can control my drinking" or "All the problems in the family are the fault of the drinker") reappear, the therapist explores these distortions in thinking and also focuses on behavior, suggesting increased meetings or contact with a sponsor. A psychodynamic approach may also be needed if Twelve-Step work opens difficulties with the Twelve-Step program itself or with other people, or if recovery unmasks unconscious unresolved conflict or issues of past trauma. If the alcoholic or family member experiences a return to pre-recovery thinking, or feels a strong upsurge in emotion, the therapist is always ready to ask: Why now? What is this about? What might be in the way of steady growth?

At this stage, the Family Recovery Guide "map" (Brown, Lewis & Liotta, 2000) can help temper discouragement as people read about what is normal in Early Recovery and see that their experiences match. Reading ahead to Ongoing Recovery imparts hope. In Early Recovery, alcoholics and family members are less out of control and impulse-driven than they were in the Transition Stage, but it is still a time of change and feeling one's way in a strange territory. Couples may feel distressed that their intimacy feels attenuated, as they lead "parallel lives until there is a stronger sense of oneself and separateness from the other" (Brown & Lewis, 1999, p. 222). Sexuality may have to be relearned without alcohol, and sexual desire of one or both partners may be greatly reduced.

The couple's distress about this, however, does not mean that the therapist's job is to focus on intimacy at this point. Distance at this stage is normal. The couple may need help to tolerate the situation as they build a new kind of intimacy based on sobriety. Recovery itself can provide the matrix for a new connection, based on a new shared reality. As Brown and Lewis point out: "The focus on alcoholism and the language that describes it [can] serve to hold partners together until they can turn their attention back to themselves as a couple" (1999, p. 221).

Besides loss of intimacy, emotional ups and downs are normative in Early Recovery, especially in the first few years. The therapist needs to understand that these fluctuations are part of normal development and do not need to be fixed. It is helpful for families, too, to know that these are normal, and, as is said in 12-Step programs, "This too shall pass." The therapist must be prepared, however, to diagnose major problems if and when they do arise in recovery, and to provide adequate treatment. For some families, the upheaval associated with Early Recovery can last for a long time–"three to five years and even longer" (Brown and Lewis, 1999, p. 223).

Feelings that arise for patients during this time need attention, but it is not a time for the therapist to initiate a focus on feelings and their historic sources. For example, if a couple chooses to put discussion of an old affair on hold, because they feel it is still too soon in their recoveries, the therapist is wise to follow their lead. Because recovery behaviors are new and often fragile, strong feelings can still lead back to drinking and other loss of control. Yet a decision not to explore old feelings and issues that are urgent or overwhelming or get in the way of recovery can also lead to relapse. It may be time to open the past, even though nobody wants to. If patients feel that they need to resolve old traumas during this time, the therapist encourages them to step up their 12-Step programs while they are dealing with these issues in therapy. Strong program involvement offers the best chance that the feelings can be contained without leading to relapse.

Practical issues also arise constantly. The Chases need help in attending to their children's needs while they themselves participate in recovery-oriented activities. They need to acknowledge that they can't be in two places at once and get help so that the children are not abandoned in the service of their recovery. Mr. and Mrs. Chase need to address Anne's drinking, Julie's occasional school refusal, and both children's loneliness and confusion. They add support for their kids by clarifying and strengthening family schedules and by trading off meeting times between them to maximize time a parent can be home with the children.

Are the Chases a recovering family if the children are having problems, including drinking? Given the behavioral and systems changes this family has experienced, the parents are now in a position to deal with their children's problems in a healthy way. They can figure out how to tighten family routines and install new sober rituals, and decide whether to get help from friends, relatives, and professionals and what kind to get. Most importantly, they can hold onto their individual recoveries. The Chase family is no longer organized by active alcoholism despite Anne's drinking. The Chases are indeed a recovering family.

The Family in Ongoing Recovery

Ongoing Recovery is the stabilization of all the change and growth that follow from acknowledging and dealing with loss of control, both for the alcoholic and for the family. It involves an understanding of the sources and consequences of one's out of control behavior. At this stage, impulses no longer lead directly to action, as thinking routinely intervenes between them. Ongoing Recovery is based on a new self awareness, as well as a new appreciation of the importance of other people, both as sources of help and support, and as separate people with their own needs, feelings, and vulnerability. A person in Ongoing Recovery, whether he believes in God or not, is in a new spiritual stance vis-a-vis the world; he realizes that he himself is not God with unlimited power, responsibility, and importance, but now sees himself as part of a larger universe.

The Chase family has now been in recovery for six years. After a period of unemployment, Mr. Chase found a new job where he receives good reviews. Mrs. Chase is working part time. They no longer go to parties during the week, but do enjoy a weekly movie date. They are feeling close to one another again in a new, deep way. They are able to have differences of opinion, and to discuss them calmly without abusing one another. Mrs. Chase's headaches are now rare. Mr. and Mrs. Chase have remained involved in their 12-Step programs, attending two to three meetings per week. Mr. Chase goes to AA before work, and Mrs. Chase attends noon meetings of Al-Anon, so that their evenings are available for their daughters. Each family member takes responsibility for one dinner per week, and Mrs. Chase does the remaining three dinners. Each family member does his or her own laundry. While the children's extra-curricular activities do not allow the family to eat together on week nights, there are family dinners on the weekend. Anne was firmly confronted about her drinking, and the parents removed all alcohol from the house. Anne had not developed a physical dependence on alcohol, and with support from her parents and her friends in Alateen was able to stop drinking. She plans to go to a local college next year. Julie continued to have school attendance problems for a few years, but now attends regularly. She goes to Alateen meetings with her sister, and both girls like being part of the family 12-Step "in-group."

The Environment. There is a fairly recent feeling of peace and order in the Chase household. People rarely raise their voices at one another, and if that does happen, it is followed by an apology. A new playfulness is sensed in the family, and people are quick to laugh at themselves. While jobs are not secure these days due to downsizing, Mr. and Mrs. Chase are both working. Mrs. Chase was successfully treated for thyroid cancer, and Mr. Chase's father died suddenly of a heart attack. While these were difficult and painful crises, the family was able to express their feelings openly and support one another through the hard times.

The System. While the family is no longer organized around drinking, the alcohol history is present in the form of recovery activities. Family members have constructed a new identity as a recovering family, and a new family "story" that includes drinking and recovery. A new ritual reinforces the organizing principle of recovery: sobriety or recovery "birthdays" are celebrated for each individual with a special dinner. Mr. and Mrs. Chase have "sponsees" of their own, newly recovering people whom they mentor in AA and Al-Anon respectively. They also are branching out and making new friends outside of their 12-Step programs. They are working on moving fluidly from self-focus to family focus and back again–the self is rarely sacrificed to the system, though all members now know how to yield in a healthy way secure in the knowledge that they also can hold their own. Mr. Chase is no longer the dominant force in the family. Mr. and Mrs. Chase are able to communicate more openly with one another, on an equal basis, and are more receptive to hearing from the children. They feel closer to each other, and have revived their sexual relationship. The family now functions without a scapegoat. Rules and boundaries are more clearly stated. The parents now act as parents, leaving the children free to challenge them openly and safely, and to participate with their peers. Anne and Julie feel safe bringing friends home, and the family is no longer isolated.

Individual Development. Mr. Chase has worked hard in his therapy on the issue of his father's alcoholism. There were upheavals with his family of origin as he learned to assert himself with his own parents. As he stayed sober, he experienced grief and mourning at the loss of his alcoholic connection with them, but he also felt a sense of freedom. Mrs. Chase focused on her tendency to ignore her needs while pleasing and deferring to others until she became overwhelmed with rage and blew up in anger. She is learning to assert herself calmly, and to acknowledge when she needs help. Working outside of the home brought with it a new self-esteem. Anne began socializing with friends from Alateen, and now has a close peer group, whose opinions are more important to her than those of her family. Julie has struggled in her therapy with low self-esteem and was prescribed antidepressants. She and her mother had a course of conjoint therapy to help Julie feel safe from attack, and less worried about her mother's ability to function. This worry had been a large part of her school refusal.

Treatment in Ongoing Recovery. Psychodynamic psychotherapy is useful in Ongoing Recovery as people feel safe enough to allow their feelings to emerge. With the behaviors of recovery firmly in place, strong feeling can now be experienced without resorting to the old coping strategies of drinking and the attitudes associated with drinking. This makes it possible to explore old sources of pain and maladaptive behavior with less threat of relapse. Now that each partner has a solid sense of self, couples therapy can help them bridge back towards intimacy.

At any point in recovery, thoughts of drinking can signal new insights or the emergence of strong feelings. These are often a sign of growth rather than impending relapse. But it is important for the therapist and the person in recovery to assess the state of recovery and any tendency toward relapse. If a recovering alcoholic talks about a real temptation to drink, or expresses feelings of omnipotence, or a belief that she can control her drinking; or if a codependent loses self focus and becomes invested in controlling other people, the therapist can return to cognitive and behavioral methods as needed, and recommend intensification of the recovery program.

MAJOR CONCLUSIONS
OF THE BROWN AND LEWIS STUDY

The stages of alcoholism recovery for the family parallel the stages of recovery for the individual alcoholic. In order for the family to be able to recover, the alcoholic family system that supported the drinking must collapse. This is extremely traumatic for the family, and things usually get worse before they get better. Families will be better able to tolerate this worsening if they understand the process of recovery, and know what is normal and what to expect. With the family system in a state of collapse, it is essential for the family to seek outside help and support in order to function. Twelve-step programs are designed to provide such support.

The therapist, too, needs to know what is normal for families going through a recovery process, in order to be able to tolerate the pain and chaos of the people in recovery. The therapist utilizes different treatment methods in different stages, including different suggestions, interpretations and interventions for different people in the same family.

- Drinking and Transition stages require an alcohol focus, using psychodynamic and cognitive methods to challenge the distorted thinking and behavior of addiction.
- Behavioral and educational approaches are most helpful in Abstinent Transition and Early Recovery to help patients learn to substitute new abstinent behaviors for the impulse to drink. Psychodynamic techniques are used in these stages only to resolve blocks to recovery movement, and not to evoke strong feeling, which could cause a relapse to active addiction.
- In Ongoing recovery, a psychodynamic method is most useful to resolve feelings that emerge in this stage, with cognitive and behavioral backup if signs of relapse emerge.

It is crucial that the needs of the children be met as much as possible during all stages of recovery. This can be a dilemma for parents who are learning for the first time in their lives to focus on themselves in a healthy way and devote time and energy to their own needs for recovery growth.

Recovery leads to long-term benefit although its path is painful and arduous. Recovery is not an end-point; it is a process of continuing change and development. It is not "happily ever after" in the sense that a recovering family has no problems. Recovery gives a family the ability to cope with life's problems both separately and together without needing to escape or lose control.

REFERENCES

Alcoholics Anonymous. (1955). New York: AA World Services.

Al-Anon Faces Alcoholism. (1984). Al-Anon Family Groups.

Bader, E., and Pearson, P. (1988). *In Quest of the Mythical Mate: A Developmental Approach to Diagnosis and Treatment in Couples Therapy.* New York: Brunner/Mazel.

Bateson, G. (1971). The cybernetics of self: A theory of alcoholism. *Psychiatry, 34*(1), pp. 1-18.

Black, C. (1981). *It Will Never Happen to Me.* Denver: MAC.

Brown, S. (1985). *Treating the Alcoholic: A Developmental Model of Recovery.* New York: Wiley.

Brown, S. (1988). *Treating Adult Children of Alcoholics: A Developmental Perspective.* New York: Wiley.

Brown, S. (1991). *Safe Passage: Recovery for Adult Children of Alcoholics.* New York: Wiley.

Brown, S. (1994). Alcoholism and trauma: A theoretical comparison and overview. *Journal of Psychoactive Drugs, 26*(4), 345-355.

Brown, S. (1995). Adult children of alcoholics: An expanded framework for assessment and diagnosis. In: S. Abbott (Ed.), *Children of Alcoholics: Selected Readings.* Rockville MD: National Association for Children of Alcoholics, pp. 41-76.

Brown, S., Beletsis, S., & Cermak, T. (1989). *Adult Children of Alcoholics in Treatment.* Orlando, FL: Health Communications.

Brown, S., & Lewis, V. (1999). *The Alcoholic Family in Recovery: A Developmental Model.* New York: Guilford Press.

Brown, S., Lewis, V., & Liotta, A. (2000). *The Family Recovery Guide: A Map for Healthy Growth.* Oakland: New Harbinger.

Cermak, T. (1986). *Diagnosing and Treating Codependence.* Minneapolis: The Johnson Institute.

Cermak, T. (1989). *A Time to Heal.* Los Angeles: Jeremy Tarcher.

Edwards, P., Harvery, C., & Whitehead, P. C. (1973). Wives of alcoholics: A critical review and analysis. *Quarterly Journal of Studies on Alcohol, 34*, pp. 651-668.

Fox, R. (1956). The alcoholic spouse. In: V. Eisenstein (Ed.), *Neurotic Interaction in Marriage.* New York: Basic Books.

Herman, J. (1992). *Trauma and Recovery.* New York: Basic Books.

Jackson, J. (1954). The adjustment of the family to the crisis of alcoholism. *Quarterly Journal of Studies on Alcoholi. 15*, pp. 562-586.

Jackson, J. (1962). Alcoholism and the family. In: D.J. Pittman, and C.R. Snyder (Eds.), *Society, Culture and Drinking Patterns,* New York: Wiley.

Jaylen Productions. (1997). *Treating Alcoholism with Stephanie Brown, Ph.D.* (video). San Francisco.

Jellinek, E. M. (1960). *The Disease Concept of Alcoholism.* New Haven, CT: College and University Press.

Khan, M. M. R. (1963). The concept of cumulative trauma. *Psychoanalytic Study of the Child, 18*, 286-306.

Krystal, H. (1978). Trauma and affects. *Psychoanalytic Study of the Child, 33*, pp. 127-152.

Nixon, K. (2006). Alcohol and adult neurogenesis: roles in neurodegeneration and recovery in chronic alcoholism. *Hippocampus, 16*(3), pp. 287-95.

Shaef, A. W. (1986). *Codependence: Misunderstood, Mistreated.* New York: Harper Collins.

Steinglass, P., Bennett, L., Wolin, S., & Reiss, D. (1987). *The Alcoholic Family.* New York: Basic Books.

Tiebout, H. (1944). Therapeutic mechanisms of Alcoholics Anonymous. *American Journal of Psychiatry, 100*, pp. 468-473.

Tiebout, H. (1953). Surrender vs. compliance in therapy with special reference to alcoholism. *Quarterly Journal of Studies on Alcohol, 14*, pp. 58-68.

Volkow, N. D., & Li, T. K. (2005). Drugs and alcohol: Treating and preventing abuse, addiction and their medical consequences. *Pharmacological Therapeutics, 108*(1), pp. 3-17.

Wolin, S., Bennett, L., & Noonan, D. (1979). Family rituals and the reoccurrence of alcoholism over generations. *American Jouranl of Psychiatry, 136*, pp. 589-593.

Wolin, S., Bennett, L., Noonan, D., & Teitelbaum, M. (1980). Disrupted family rituals. *Journal of Studies on Alcohol, 41*, 199-214.

doi:10.1300/J020v26n01_03

Family Behavior Loop Mapping:
A Technique to Analyze the Grip
Addictive Disorders Have on Families
and to Help Them Recover

Michael R. Liepman, MD
Roberto Flachier, PhD
Ruqiya Shama Tareen, MD

SUMMARY. A family systems therapy technique applied to families suffering from chronic addictive disorders has been developed to document graphically information from a detailed behavioral analysis of family interactions. In a family interview, a step-by-step description of thoughts,

---

Michael R. Liepman is Clinical Professor of Psychiatry and Director of Psychiatry Research at Michigan State University College of Human Medicine, Kalamazoo Center for Medical Studies (MSU/KCMS) and Adjunct Professor in the Specialty Program on Alcohol & Drug Abuse (SPADA) of Western Michigan University College of Health and Human Services. He is Medical Director of the Jim Gilmore Jr. Community Healing Center.

Roberto Flachier is Clinical Assistant Professor of Psychiatry at MSU/KCMS and Adjunct Associate Professor in the Department of Psychology at Western Michigan University.

Ruqiya Shama Tareen is Clinical Assistant Professor of Psychiatry at MSU/KCMS.

Address correspondence to: Michael R. Liepman MD, MSU/KCMS Psychiatry, 1722 Shaffer Street, Suite 3, Kalamazoo, MI 49048-1633 (E-mail: Liepman@kcms.msu.edu).

This article is dedicated in loving memory to Loretta Y. Silvia, PhD, whose collaboration, encouragement and ideas helped formulate the conceptual framework on which this manuscript is based.

[Haworth co-indexing entry note]: "Family Behavior Loop Mapping: A Technique to Analyze the Grip Addictive Disorders Have on Families and to Help Them Recover." Liepman, Michael R., Roberto Flachier, and Ruqiya Shama Tareen. Co-published simultaneously in *Alcoholism Treatment Quarterly* (The Haworth Press) Vol. 26, No. 1/2, 2008, pp. 59-80; and: *Family Intervention in Substance Abuse: Current Best Practices* (ed: Oliver J. Morgan, and Cheryl H. Litzke) The Haworth Press, 2008, pp. 59-80. Single or multiple copies of this article are available for a fee from The Haworth Document Delivery Service [1-800-HAWORTH, 9:00 a.m. - 5:00 p.m. (EST). E-mail address: docdelivery@haworthpress.com].

feelings and actions of each family member is sought which is then drawn as a flow diagram for the therapist and family to study together. Contrasts between the thoughts, feelings and actions associated with episodes of using intoxicants versus abstinence facilitates crafting a mutually acceptable solution for the family that can be diagrammed, enacted and practiced. The theoretical basis for this approach is reviewed and the technique is described. Applications to other mental and medical disorders that have a chronic relapsing nature are suggested. *doi:10.1300/J020v26n01_04 [Article copies available for a fee from The Haworth Document Delivery Service: 1-800-HAWORTH. E-mail address: <docdelivery@haworthpress.com> Website: <http://www.HaworthPress.com> © 2008 by The Haworth Press. All rights reserved.]*

KEYWORDS. Addiction, alcohol-other drug treatment, family therapy, family systems, behavioral analysis, behavior chain, stages of change, motivational interviewing

PROLOGUE

Even as good shone upon the countenance of the one, evil was written broadly and plainly on the face of the other . . . all human beings, as we meet them, are commingled out of good and evil . . . and Edward Hyde, alone in the ranks of mankind, was pure evil. . . . At that time my virtue slumbered; my evil, kept awake by ambition, was alert and swift to seize the occasion; and the thing that was projected was Edward Hyde . . . Hence, although I had now two characters as well as two appearances, one was wholly evil, and the other was still the old Henry Jekyll, that incongruous compound of whose reformation and improvement I had already learned to despair. . . . The movement was thus wholly toward the worse.

(Robert Louis Stevenson, 1886)

INTRODUCTION

It was a complete mystery why Dr. Henry Jekyll, esteemed scientist and physician, would associate himself with the likes of Mr. Edward Hyde, a mean, despicable person prone to wanton violence and disregard for the personal rights of others. But both men cloaked themselves in a veil of secrecy in Dr. Jekyll's home to protect their mysterious activities from prying eyes. As we read on in the novel, we discover that both men shared the same body, taking turns as to who was in control at any particular time. Driven initially by curiosity, and later by an irrepressible urge to once again experience the thrill of the transformation and to study it scientifically, each time he drank the powerful potion, Dr. Henry Jekyll's identity shifted to that of his alter ego, Edward Hyde. Only after the intoxication wore off would he return to his usual self, having to worry about what Hyde had done while under the influence of the mysterious chemical.

It also is a mystery why perfectly decent human beings known in the community for their good works, talents, and kindness towards others suddenly change their ways to become selfish, inconsiderate, and shameful. Once in treatment for their addictive diseases, these persons return to their prior selves with all their charm and high values. But the mystery becomes even more vexing when, after leaving treatment, with the encouragement of their loved ones, they relinquish sobriety in short order returning to their despicable selves once again despite all the fine promises they had made to us, their treatment professionals, their families, and even themselves (Steinglass, Davis, & Berenson, 1977).

In this paper we will introduce a way to understand relapse behavior in addiction in the context of the family system. We will show how to assess and document the interactions that lead up to and through relapses. We will show how to compare *pros* and *cons* of abstinence and of relapse at the conceptual level of the family system to demonstrate a reason why family members often engage in supportive and/or hostile enabling behaviors that encourage and assist the chemically dependent person to relapse. We will then show how to design an alternative set of interactions that is likely to eliminate or reduce the frequency of relapses to intoxicant use by the addicted person and to codependent enabling behaviors by the rest of the family. Finally we will suggest some other applications of this procedure to other chronic, recurring conditions.

WHEN INTOXICANT USE BECOMES A PROBLEM FOR FAMILIES

The use of intoxicants usually begins mildly with teen experimentation and then over months to years, the behavior gradually evolves into one of greater intensity or risk with impaired function (Liepman, Keller, Botelho, Monroe, & Sloane, 1998). In some families, addiction problems recur over generations. Just when someone in the family first realizes that addiction is a problem is difficult to predict or describe. Nonetheless, usually this does not happen early in the process.

During the pre-recovery phase of addiction disorders, the intoxicated person's behavior begets complementary responses from bystanders. For example, if an intoxicated mother fails to make dinner, her teenage daughter may cook dinner for the family. This enables mom to drink tomorrow without worries of her family going hungry. Repeated episodes train the bystanders to repeat these coping responses to the intoxicated person's irresponsible behavior. Adaptation to the addict's dysfunctional behavior and drug-induced personality and behavior changes alters the family's behavioral repertoire. In the example, the daughter develops confidence and self-esteem in her new role as surrogate mother, while reassuring the family that they will never have to go without dinner even when mom is drinking, and while reassuring mom that her drinking is not that serious of a problem for the family (Koppel, Stimmler, & Perone, 1980; Levinson & Ashenberg-Straussner, 1978; Liepman, 1993).

Alcoholic males at least 6 months into recovery and their committed female partners were surveyed on their impressions of their family interactions and sexual function, contrasting between abstinent and drinking conditions. The results showed dramatic shifts in function from quite pathological in the drinking condition to quite normative in the abstinent condition (Liepman, Nirenberg et al., 1989; Nirenberg, Liepman et al., 1990). However, quite remarkably, 17 of the 20 couples scored at least one dimension of their responses on the McMaster Family Assessment Device (FAD) in the reverse polarity indicating that at least one dimension improved in the drinking condition and worsened with abstinence (Liepman et al., 1990, 1993). All twenty couples responded to at least 4 (range: 4-21 out of 120) items on the FAD in which the more healthy responses were associated with the drinking condition. The alcoholics and their partners responded this way on 1-23 items and 1-18 items of 60, respectively (Liepman & Nirenberg, in preparation). While the specific function(s) that improved with drinking or deteriorated with abstinence varied from one couple to the next, there was a consistent impression that the drinking served to normalize something for each of these families making it difficult to bear persistent sobriety and easy to welcome relapse.

Thus, when treatment and early recovery begins, whenever intoxicant use ceases, these families experience a mixture of improvements in some aspects of function but a deterioration of certain other key interactions within the family. If they discover that relapse can improve this latter aspect of their relationship, then it makes sense that the addicted person would dutifully resume use of intoxicants for the benefit of the family. Quite curious but understandable, the spouse, children, and significant others also may behave in ways that are likely to enable or provoke a relapse in order to relieve this sort of tension within the family system (Frankenstein, Hay, & Nathan, 1985; Jacob, Ritchey, Cvitkovic, & Blane, 1981; Steinglass et al., 1977). In essence, what they are doing is utilizing the flexibility their family possesses by virtue of its ability to oscillate between the abstinent condition and the intoxication condition as needed. In contrast, those of us in the treatment professions ask and expect these families to diminish their family flexibility by maintaining continuous abstinence and ceasing all enabling behavior, no matter how uncomfortable that makes them feel!

Greater flexibility in families confers greater durability while greater rigidity may lead to family dysfunction or fragmentation (Minuchin, 1974). If addiction treatment robs a family of flexibility, the likelihood of relapse or emergence of other pathology increases. The Cycle of Family Function (Smilkstein, 1980) asserts that a family can remain stable in a pathological equilibrium in which bad things such as chronic intoxicant abuse are accepted by the family as a means to maintain family stability. However, a severe stressful event can disrupt this solution leading to a variety of outcomes: (1) the family can find effective help to achieve healthy family equilibrium through recovery; (2) the family can fail to find effective help and can slip back into pathological equilibrium; or (3) the family can fracture and dissolve or eject a member. What may make the difference in outcomes would be the available internal family resources (i.e., within the nuclear and extended family) and external resources (i.e., community agencies, health care providers, which could include an astute family therapist), and which of these choices the family members are willing to pursue.

It must be emphasized that much of what happens during enabling behavior is motivated by a desire to be helpful, supportive, nurturing and loving towards the addicted person. Enabling of the supportive variety unfortunately and paradoxically makes it easier for the addiction to progress without the restraints of responsibilities, obligations, social expectations, even rules (Black, 2001; Liepman, Wolper, & Vazquez, 1982). Enablers run interference for the addicted person against the world of reality by making alibis, covering up, lying, paying off debts, taking up the slack, diverting attention, and telling them how much they are loved and cared about in spite of the negative impacts the addiction is having on those who care about them. Often enablers undermine one another or even fight amongst themselves over the addicted person, and they often lie to and conceal things from each other to make the impact of their loved one's addictive disorder appear less severe than it really is. Their behavior makes it easier for the addicted person to continue to stay ill and to resist pressures to quit (Liepman, 1993).

As addiction progresses to the point of bringing more serious harm to the family, some of the positive, loving feelings may be replaced by resentful, angry feelings which may motivate directing aggressive behavior towards the addicted person (Gorman & Rooney, 1979). At this point it may become apparent, inside the family and to outsiders, that the harmful behavior is associated with an addiction disorder. Bystanders feel anger and resentment over helplessness they experience when the addicted person does not seek help as suggested or the disorder does not respond to family efforts to "help them get better" or to "straighten up" or to seek treatment, or when treatment efforts are abandoned and relapse ensues. Often they become increasingly hostile towards the addicted person, using sarcasm, yelling, name calling, threats, and even violence to express their anger. They may run away from home, pursue infidelity, invest heavily in work or school or other activities, or alternatively they may begin to abuse intoxicants. Hostile enabling behaviors provide the addicted person with an excuse for retreating to intoxicants. Research has demonstrated that hostility expressed towards alcoholics *increases* relapse frequency and severity (O'Farrell, Hooley, Fals-Stewart, & Cutter, 1998).

READINESS TO CHANGE

Prochaska's revolutionary concept asserts that people change their behavior as the result of a process involving several consecutive *stages of change* beginning at *denial* [precontemplation], progressing to *ambivalence* [contemplation], then *getting ready to change* [preparedness], then moving to *readiness to change* [decision], then the actual *change* [behavior change], and *maintenance* of that change [relapse prevention] (Prochaska & DiClemente, 1986). This model can be extended by adding *denial of relapse* [precontemplation of relapse], *ambivalence about relapse* [contemplation of relapse], *readiness to relapse*, actual *relapse* behavior, and *maintenance of relapse* [which in essence is precontemplation of recovery] back at the start.

When considering the isolated individual with an addiction disorder, this process is fairly straightforward and can be positively influenced by

Motivational Interviewing (Miller & Rollnick, 1991). In addition to motivation, self-efficacy and self-confidence are important ingredients needed for the individual to change. Treatment in residential and outpatient addiction recovery programs along with ongoing support from 12-step or other recovery support groups can assist individuals to achieve and maintain abstinence from alcohol and other drugs. It is clear from empirical research that use of treatment strategies specific to the stage of readiness to change is a key ingredient for engagement in treatment and for successful treatment outcome (DiClemente et al., 1991; Martin, Velicer, & Fava, 1996).

However, part of the psychoeducation of treatment and support groups emphasizes warning the newly recovering person to distance him/herself from toxic relationships with people who continue to use chemicals or who enable or encourage substance use. This is easier to do when the toxic relationships are with friends or casual acquaintances rather than with one's own family. While family may provide lip-service for the idea of getting sober, it is common for relatives inadvertently to provoke or encourage relapse by their words or deeds. Sneaking drugs into detox, asking the relative to leave treatment prematurely for some reason, celebrating sobriety with a drink, tempting the newly sober person to test his/her commitment to sobriety, complaining about how much time is spent at 12-step groups, being jealous about new friendships made there, or provoking a relapse by hostility are examples of ways that families collude with the disease against sobriety by triggering relapse. This may explain why the rate of relapse is so high when the addicted person returns home and why family involvement in treatment and aftercare are so helpful in improving outcome (Copello, Velleman, & Templeton, 2005; Edwards & Steinglass, 1995; Stanton & Shadish, 1997).

When a substance abuser is ready to change, there is no guarantee that the relatives (enablers) are ready as well, and vice versa. In fact, a parent, partner, child or sibling may not have the self-efficacy, the confidence, or the will to promote positive change. What is worse, they may subconsciously wish for relapse to occur as a means to temporarily *solve* other problems of the family, and recovery might actually be perceived as a threat to the family. Thus, the addicted person and family members may be in different motivational stages regarding whether treatment ought to occur and succeed. Getting them all on the same page in synchrony poses a major challenge for treatment providers and family therapists.

It is this manner of thinking that spawned the notion of creating a family interview to assess both the family advantages and disadvantages of both abstinence *and* relapse. The interview seeks to contrast the abstinent intervals with intoxicated intervals in terms of pros and cons as reflected in the interactions between family members. Perhaps because of our stated goal to prevent relapse, many families do not naturally admit to a clinician the advantages of relapse and disadvantages of abstinence. This is assessed through a step-by-step *behavioral chain analysis* (Linehan, 1993) wherein each element of the interactions is documented in graphic form to tease out the individual contributions to the sequence of events that transpire within the family as the cycle unfolds. As they perceive the pros and cons before them, the family can better understand why members make the decisions they do. If the entire family is present for the interview, they can develop better mutual understanding and synchronize their efforts to initiate and support recovery.

"Relapse is a process rather than an event" (Gorski, 1989; Marlatt & Gordon, 1985). Relapse is a series of steps taken by the alcoholic or addict just prior to beginning to resume use of intoxicants after an interval of abstinence. The sequence of steps in the oft recurring process can be documented including the feelings, thoughts and behaviors of the substance abuser, and we broaden the analysis by documenting those of the enablers/victims from the family (or significant others). Once these are documented in sequence on a visual map, an examination focusing on the contrasts between the two parts (the abstinent portion vs. the intoxicants use portion) of the map usually reveals blatant differences among which can be found both advantages and disadvantages of relapse to the family system (Liepman, Silvia, & Nirenberg, 1989; Silvia & Liepman, 1991a).

DEVISING A CORRECTIVE MAP

Once a map of family interactions reveals the incentives for relapse, a corrective map can be devised. It is the advantages of relapse and disadvantages of abstinence that are the focus of correction. This is a creative process in which the therapist and the family together devise a way to take an *advantage of relapse* and moving it to the abstinent side of the map; that is, by finding a way to create this advantage in the abstinent condition. This step is critical in helping the family to enhance its function during sobriety and simultaneously to remove the unique value of relapse so that the negative consequences unopposed by advantages can serve as a natural deterrent to future relapse. (This will be demonstrated in an example below.) Once moved on the map, the change must be enacted by the family and practiced a few times until it becomes self-reinforcing.

Doing the Family Behavior Loop Map (FBLM) Interview

A FBLM interview can be done in an hour or two, integrated into whatever model of family therapy one prefers. It is best done with the whole nuclear family present, but the information often can be obtained with fewer members of the family participating. However, reduced representation at the interview will diminish the accuracy and richness of the data obtained. The synchronization of recovery efforts among family members also may be lost. Although small children are not likely to contribute verbally to the process, their presence may demonstrate observable family interactive behavior. Latency aged children and teens may easily contribute verbally. Sometimes significant others or extended family members who spend a lot of time with the family may have interesting information to add to the interview.

The founders of this process began with slate chalkboards or paper flipcharts on which to draw the map, but recent technological advances such as dry erase boards, sticky notes, and computers have made the process easier. To begin, the therapist(s) or interviewer(s) should draw a horizontal line bisecting the page/board/screen. Above the line is labeled *not using* or *abstinent* and below the line is labeled *using [drugs or alcohol]*.

The process is then explained to the participants. They are told that we are seeking the stepwise sequence of events that occur before and after the transition from the abstinent condition to drinking/drug use and the transition back. The purpose of this assessment is to better understand how the family participates in the process of the transitions with the possibility of helping the family to learn different ways to react that might reduce the frequency and the duration of relapses. Ask the family members not to talk all at once, but to make sure that we have an accurate picture of what goes on so that the final product is useful to them.

Have someone choose a recent relapse to use as an example. This will still be fresh in everyone's memory and can serve as a template for the overall pattern of relapses. Later on, other examples can be brought up to see how similar they are to the one already elucidated. Frequently they will be quite similar with perhaps only small details being different. However, in some families an entirely different sequence of events may be described representing a completely different loop on the map. Sometimes a loop will branch at a certain point at which the sequence diverges from what already has been documented; later in the sequence it may merge again with the documented loop at a particular point.

The display should be legible and easily visible to all participants so that they can help to edit it as it evolves. Make it clear to all participants that it is preferred that they speak up if they notice inaccuracies or incomplete renditions of what actually goes on at home. Promptly give compliments to each family member when he or she makes a contribution to elucidating the sequence of events. As there usually is a need for multiple corrections and adjustments in the diagram, the more forgiving media such as sticky notes or dry erase boards or computer displays are less messy and easier to revise. Frequently icons and arrows must be moved around to accommodate inserted intermediate steps or branches.[1]

Icons

Three different shapes of figures (icons: see Table 1) are used to represent thoughts, feelings and actions (behaviors). This makes it easier to keep track of the process. It reminds us that thoughts and feelings are different, and that they typically are found in response to behaviors

TABLE 1. Icons Used in FBL Maps

Rectangle	Bill: *Sally always gets her way*	Thoughts
Diamond	Bill is sad, then angry	Feelings emotions or somatic sensations
Oval	Bill yells at Sally	Actions (Behavior)
Arrow		Next step in process
Partial Sequence	Bill: Sally always gets her way / Bill yells at Sally / Bill is sad, then angry / Sally is scared, then angry	Temporal sequence of a series of events in the family dance

of others and lead to behaviors in self. The best FBL Maps include not only the sequence of behaviors but also the intervening thoughts and feelings.

Inside each icon one writes a brief description of the action/thought/feeling. The level of specificity may vary and may be altered as the FBL Map evolves. Typical examples of feelings are listed in Table 2.

The thoughts and behaviors are too variable to limit to a table. In general, thoughts may include expectation, observation, perception, attribution, interpretation, decision, thoughts about craving, a plan, or others. Thoughts can be put inside the icons as quotes such as, for example: Bill (interpretation): *"I think I'm in trouble with Sally,"* or Mary (thought about craving): *"This would be a good time for some wine."* Using different colors of sticky notes or markers or computer icons for each person in the family helps distinguish the icons to keep them straight.

Arrows

Arrows connect steps in the process (icons) as they are described to occur in a temporal sequence. Arrows may connect a thought to a feeling or vice versa and then another arrow may connect a thought to a behavior. Arrows may connect the behavior of one person to the thoughts (perception) of another. In this way the interactions of family members can be mapped out for visual inspection and analysis. As some

TABLE 2. Feelings

Basic Feeling	Other words representing variations on basic feeling
Anger	Annoyed, Upset, Irritated, Furious, Enraged
Fear	Worried, Anxious, Nervous, Scared, Terrified
Sadness	Unhappy, Disappointed, Grieving, Distraught, Ashamed
Happiness	Satisfied, Pleased, Delighted, Excited, Euphoric
Craving	Hungry, urge to drink, smoke, or use drugs
Sexual arousal	Horny, Wanting sexual interaction or activity
Sexual aversion	Desire to be left alone, not approached or touched
Physical discomfort or sensations	Itchy, Pain/Sore, Hot, Cold, Nauseated, Tired, Weak, Urge to urinate or move bowels or sneeze or vomit, Pain in vagina, Taste in mouth

interpersonal interactions are mutual and complex, two-sided arrows may best represent these interactions.

Sequences

Starting usually just before crossing a line and working in both directions, forwards and backwards, one gradually elucidates the steps that occur by placing icons connected by arrows. If one began with the events proximal to a relapse when intoxicant use began, one can follow the chain of events until the use of intoxicants stops again. Or, one can skip to the events leading to cessation of intoxicant use (crossing back over the line into the abstinent condition) and elucidate those. Then one can connect both fragments of the chain of events to form a loop by filling in what happens in between.

Loops

When a series of arrows and icons form a closed circle (called a loop), one can follow the *family dance* around and around, assuring the therapist and family that they have captured the essence of a chronic, recurring process. Usually there will be more than one loop drawn on a map. Branch points represent choices or options for responses that can generate different paths for the sequence to follow. Like in a dance, there may be variations in the sequence of the steps. There are three types of loops: (1) Some of the loops may avoid intoxicant use; on the map, the entire loop will stay on the abstinent side of the line that bisects the map separating abstinence from intoxicant use. These loops may provide some insight as to how the family maintains abstinence for periods of time. (2) Some loops may be entirely on the intoxicated side of the bisecting line. These loops represent conditions that support continuing use of intoxicants and indicate how chronic binges are sustained. (3) Some loops may cross the bisecting line from abstinent to intoxicated and back again. These loops will be most helpful in discovering the advantages and disadvantages of relapse and of abstinence. Within these loops will be shifts in behaviors, thoughts and feelings, and relationships between members of the family will change. Power, prestige, respect, leadership, happiness, anger, disappointment, self-esteem, shame, aggressiveness or dominance, mutuality, insecurity, expressiveness, honesty or dishonesty may oscillate from one person to another repeatedly as the family dances through the loop.

Once the map is nearly complete, it is wise to examine the process described by the map to see if it makes sense as drawn. One can choose any location on the map to begin, and then follow the sequence of events all the way around the cycle to make certain it is described accurately. This should be done with the family so they can correct inaccuracies and make suggestions for alterations. When there are multiple loops, one should follow each of the loops all the way back to the beginning. Sequences of events that do not form a complete loop should be finished–there must be some missing steps (and information) if they do not form full loops.

When documenting the map, it may come to pass that several loops are present that seem rather similar in their character. One should look carefully at the choices of words written inside the icons. If there are some common features, it is acceptable to generalize the words in the icons so that the duplicate loops can be superimposed or merged into one. This tends to simplify the map, making it easier to understand and work with when devising a corrective map.

It is not uncommon for one member to be cast in the role of the bad person (scapegoat) in the family, being blamed for all that goes wrong (Black, 2001; Wegscheider-Cruse, 1989). Often, the family blames the addict, and sometimes the addict will become defensive and blame others in the family or someone outside the family for causing a relapse or continuation of use. Often family members, especially the spouse and children, blame themselves for the relapse. It is extremely important that by mapping the detailed steps of family interactions, each member of the family can see his/her own contributions to the complex interplay of thoughts, feelings and actions that make up the whole *family dance*. This takes away the pejorative element since each step is a reaction to the previous one and leads to the next one. It becomes clear to the therapist *and* the family that they are simply caught up in a cyclical, systemic, interactive process in which no single member is the entire cause or the victim. Hence, with a sigh of relief, each member can lower his/her defenses and cooperate in finding a solution together in synchrony. The challenge is to find a way to change the family dance to one that causes less unpleasantness and harm and brings more joy and satisfaction to their lives. It also introduces more sense of control over a process that previously seemed to elude control. The family therapy concept of *balance of therapist allegiance* between each member of the family and the rule to *stop the blaming,* both important for family therapists to apply in working with families, are consistent with this model.

Searching for Benefits of the Intoxicant Use Portion of the Map

Visual inspection of the map should suggest the secondary gain of the intoxicated portion of the map. How does this portion of the map benefit the family in such a way that the family would repeatedly trade risk of harm in order to obtain this benefit? Compare the positive elements *for the family as a whole* from each side of the line that bisects the map. There should be something positive on the intoxicated side of the map that is valuable to the family that is missing from the abstinent side of the map. If not, it is doubtful that the family would endure the negative aspects without some gain to counterbalance it.

Assuming that this could be subconsciously rather than consciously known, do not expect the family members to supply this for you on a silver platter; however, if one shows it to the family, they may be able to acknowledge its veracity. Often family members will remark that everything on the map they already knew, but they never saw it put together in that way and that it fits their family quite well.

CASE EXAMPLE: BILL AND SALLY

Bill and Sally are married. Both have been marijuana smokers since college when they first met. They typically smoke pot in the evening after the children have gone to bed to relax and to get in the mood for sex. They both believe that pot smoking is necessary to calm their nerves from the stress of their work days and home life. Both Bill and Sally have quite a temper. Sally is moody, especially around her menstrual periods. Bill tends to get mad whenever he does not get his way. By the time they are ready for bed, they usually have been fighting for a couple of hours.

Bill has been attempting to recover from an alcohol problem now for several years. He joined AA two years ago after completing a residential treatment triggered by threats of divorce from Sally after his second drunk driving arrest occurred with the children in the car. The Child Protective Services (CPS) threatened to take the children from their parents unless Bill entered treatment, and they permitted his return to the home only after receiving good reports from his AA sponsor and his counselor and three months of breath testing negative for alcohol. Since that time, he has resumed drinking briefly for a day or less on several occasions. He has not returned to counseling or residential treatment.

His AA attendance varies, but without question it has reduced in frequency from the days when he was under the tight scrutiny of CPS. His seriousness and honesty at AA are less than optimal. He is not currently taking any medication to curb his craving or deter drinking. His and Sally's pot smoking has never been addressed in counseling, AA meetings, or conversations with his sponsor as they fear CPS sanctions should the truth get out. Figure 1 shows the drinking loop with the payoff of separation to provide relief of anger and aggression. Sally seeks nurturance from her children, and Bill seeks nurturance from drinking buddies and his mother.

Figure 2 shows a loop of their dysfunctional interactions involving smoking marijuana and yelling at one another. Examine the map carefully to see how the sequence of events leads to the interactions described. The positive element in this map is that they are able to be affectionate with one another after smoking marijuana together. Also, the marijuana smoking helps them to resolve their conflict. However, it does not facilitate washing the dishes or amicably solving other problems.

Prescribing Alternate Loops or Correcting Dysfunctional Loops

The identified loop(s) that serve(s) the family in some important way, thus creating ambivalence as it is simultaneously both helpful and harmful to the family, must either be extinguished or altered in such a way that it no longer enters the intoxicant use portion of the map. The challenge is to create an acceptable alternative way of achieving this same advantage without needing to have the addicted person become intoxicated and the family to have to suffer the consequences. In other words, there should be an alternative loop that avoids the intoxicant use portion of the map, yet that benefits the family in a similar manner to the advantage that was found in the intoxicant use arm of the loop that we hope to extinguish.

In some cases there is a loop that already exists in the family dance repertoire that stays entirely on the abstinent side of the map that can be modified to make it more beneficial to the family. One of these loops can be reinforced to make it become the preferred way of reacting. This is analogous to a detour in the road that previously was less traveled but that becomes more traveled because something is blocking the main road. If not already present when making corrective maps, sober alternative loops may be artificially constructed by negotiating with the family to try something different that might suffice to achieve the advantages

FIGURE 1. Alcohol loop of Family Behavior Loop Map on Bill and Sally. **A** represents the point at which Sally alienates Bill by her aggressive attacks—she initiates and reinforces a schism between them. **B** shows where her posttraumatic stress disorder is triggered by the odor of alcohol on Bill's breath. She initially feels nauseated, then recalls her abusive Dad. **C** is when Bill provides self-relief of dysphoria by drinking or escape to enablers. **D** represents the advantages of this loop. Temporary separation provides a break for each to cool down before they resume proximity. Bill is represented by gray icons and Sally by white icons.

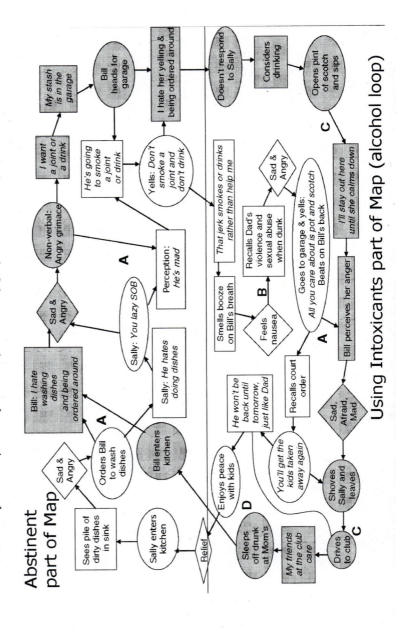

FIGURE 2. Cannabis loop of Family Behavior Loop Map on Bill and Sally. **A** represents the point at which Sally alienates Bill by her aggressive attacks–she initiates a schism between them. **B** Bill accepts the schism by seeking an escape. **C** indicates when Sally realizes she is losing Bill, and she tries to abort his escape to the garage, but only alienates him more with the same aggressive tactics. **D** points out when Sally rejoins her husband in the garage in an effort to draw him back into the interaction. **E** shows Bill reconnecting with Sally by offering her a joint. **F** shows the payoff of mutual intimacy that was not present in the prickly abstinent part of the map. **G** shows their return to the kitchen with the same dirty dishes in the sink–the same unresolved problem remains available to send them on another cycle through the map. Note that this loop is more reinforcing for the couple at **F** than the alcohol loop.

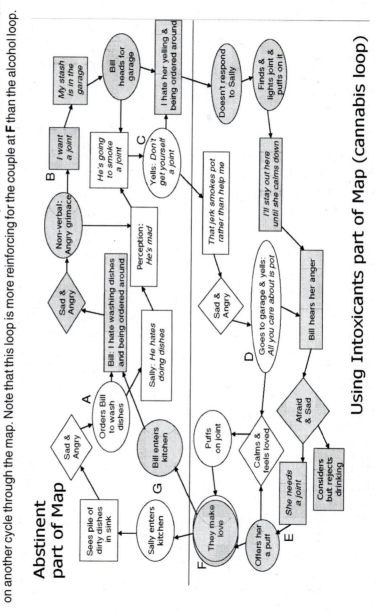

Abstinent part of Map

Using Intoxicants part of Map (cannabis loop)

formerly provided by a relapse without actually taking intoxicants. If the new loop is truly well designed and effectively provides the same advantages (without the down side) that previously were only attained by using intoxicants, the negative consequences of relapse will effectively extinguish the old loop of behavior. The new or corrected loop must not cause harm to any member of the family and it must provide benefit to each member *via helping the whole family* without invoking the need for use of intoxicants.

The new loop must be clearly delineated for the family so that they can try to enact it. They might benefit from rehearsing it in the presence of the therapist, or at least running through it verbally. It should be documented visually on paper so that the family can take it home with them. Also, recommendations on how to avoid entering any of the loops that formerly led to relapse should be provided. It is important to elicit the family's commitment to try the new loop; each member should be clear on his/her role and agree to try that preferentially at the next opportunity. All members should commit to encourage one another to enact the new loop at the appropriate time and to bring back to the next therapy session clear notes on how it went and what happened. When they return, their collective feedback on the pros and cons of the new loop should be reviewed. If there are rough spots, fine tuning can be done by making minor changes to the new loop. If they had difficulty employing the new loop, perhaps major changes will be necessary. As with any treatment for addiction, use of recovery support groups, individual, group and family counseling and anti-craving medications should be integrated into the loops and be reinforced.

Example of Discovering Advantages and Prescribing an Alternative Healthy Loop for Sally and Bill

The sequence of events starts to go awry when Sally orders Bill to wash the dishes, a task he hates (see Figures 1 and 2). The aggressive way Sally communicates with Bill adds to his anger. She could approach this in a much more diplomatic fashion by saying perhaps: *Hon, let's see if together we can knock off the dishes quickly so we can do other things we enjoy later. Do you prefer to wash or to dry the dishes?* (see Figure 3). By offering to help Bill with the dishes, she levels the playing field in terms of power in the relationship and reduces the size and unpleasantness of the task. By saying it assertively (*asking: let us do the dishes together* rather than *ordering: you do them alone*), she makes it a team effort which is consistent with assertive communication

FIGURE 3. Corrective loop for Bill and Sally to move sexual intimacy into, and to remove aggressive conflict behavior from the abstinent portion of the map. **A** shows new, assertive behavior by Sally where she uses affection rather than hostility to enlist Bill to help her wash dishes. **B** shows Bill responding to her initiative with kindness and interest. **C** points out the payoff of intimacy in the abstinent condition. Since the dishes are done, it will take another meal before the dirty dishes reappear in the sink. No need for pot-smoking or drinking and escape to resolve the schism. Note that the loop does not cross the "using intoxicants" line.

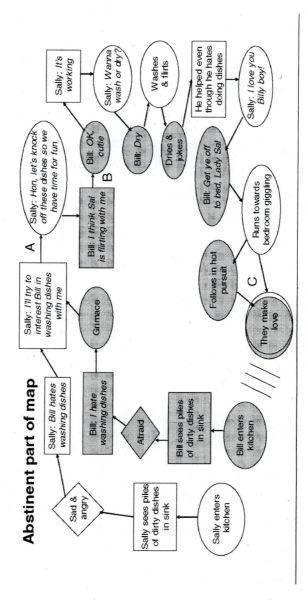

Abstinent part of map

Using intoxicants part of map

77

and good family relations. Bill is much less likely to feel demoted to dishwasher. He can get some quality talk time with Sally while helping her with the dishes. Each feels better because the partner is helping. Both will appreciate the empty sink and clean dishes when they finish the job. By adding a flirtatious tone as she suggests benefits of completing the unpleasant task quickly, Sally makes Bill more receptive and sets the tone for a happy ending for both of them.

After the hostile non-verbal interchange between them at the outset in the dysfunctional loop (Figures 1 and 2), they go off in their own separate ways until Bill relapses either to alcohol or cannabis use. Bill quells his anger by using intoxicants. In Figure 2, he offers Sally a joint to quell her anger. He reinforces their pattern of achieving sexual intimacy by smoking together. By practicing civility and assertive interactions (Figure 3), Bill and Sally can stay together throughout the entire interchange without having to relapse (use intoxicants). They come to appreciate each other and need not drink nor smoke marijuana to express affection or to resolve conflicts.

For more examples of FBL maps and their corresponding corrective maps, see (Liepman, Silvia, & Nirenberg, 1989; Silvia & Liepman, 1991a). For a video of the procedure, see (Silvia & Liepman, 1991b).

APPLICATION TO OTHER DISORDERS

It is likely that this procedure also can be used to analyze the loops of family interactions with other oscillating disorders that have an emotional or behavioral component. These disorders must be episodic and recurrent such as asthma, diabetic ketoacidosis, migraines, peptic ulcers, ulcerative colitis, anorexia or bulimia nervosa, domestic violence, depression, bipolar disorder, schizophrenia, gambling or sexual addiction. We have found no published data to support this impression nor have we developed any anecdotal evidence that this is true, but we challenge clinicians working with these families to look as well for similar positive value in the illness phase of these oscillating conditions.

NOTE

1. A software product is under development by the first author to facilitate using this technique on computers.

REFERENCES

Black, C. (2001). It will never happen to me, 2nd edition. Bainbridge Island, WA: MAC Publishing.

Copello, AG, Velleman, RDB, & Templeton LJ. (2005). Family interventions in the treatment of alcohol and drug problems. *Drug & Alcohol Rev 24:*369-85.

DiClemente, CC, Prochaska, JO, Fairhurst, SK, Velicer, WF, Velasquez, MM, & Rossi, JS. (1991). The process of smoking cessation: An analysis of precontemplation, contemplation, and preparation stages of change. *J Consult Clin Psychol 59:*295-304.

Edwards, ME, & Steinglass, P. (1995). Family therapy treatment outcomes for alcoholism. *Journal of Marital and Family Therapy 21:*475-509.

Frankenstein, W, Hay, WM, & Nathan, PE. (1985). Effects of intoxication on alcoholics' marital communication and problem solving. *J Studies on Alcohol 46:*1-6.

Gorman, JM, & Rooney, JF. (1979). Delay in seeking help and onset of crises among Al-Anon wives. *Amer J Drug & Alcohol Abuse 6:*223-33.

Gorski, TT. (1989). Passages through recovery: An action plan for preventing relapse. Centre City, MN: Hazelden.

Jacob, T, Ritchey, D, Cvitkovic, JF, & Blane, HT. (1981). Communication styles of alcoholic and nonalcoholic families when drinking and not drinking. *J Studies on Alcohol 42:*466-82.

Koppel, F, Stimmler, L, & Perone, F. (1980). The enabler: A motivational tool in treating the alcoholic. *Social Casework 61:*577-580.

Levinson, VR, & Ashenberg-Straussner, SL. (1978). Social workers as "enablers" in the treatment of alcoholics. *Social Casework 59:*14-20.

Liepman, MR. (1993). Using family influence to motivate alcoholics to enter treatment: The Johnson Institute Intervention Approach. In TJ O'Farrell Ed. *Marital and Family Therapy in AlcoholismTreatment* (pp. 54-77). New York: Guilford.

Liepman, MR, Keller, DM, Botelho, R, Monroe, AD, & Sloane, MA. (1998). Preventing substance abuse by adolescents: A guide for primary care clinicians. In PJ Fahey, RT Brown, LL Gabel Eds. *Primary Care: Clinics in Office Practice: Adolescent Medicine.* Philadelphia: WB Saunders.

Liepman, MR, & Nirenberg, TD. (In preparation). Drinking is better than sobriety in certain ways: Responses to questionnaires by alcoholic men and their female partners about drinking and abstaining.

Liepman, MR, Nirenberg, TD, Doolittle, RH, Begin, AM, Broffman, TE, & Babich, M. (1989). Family functioning of male alcoholics and their female partners during periods of drinking and abstinence. *Family Process 28:*239-49.

Liepman, MR, Nirenberg, TD, Doolittle, RH, Broffman, TE, & Silvia, LY. November (1993). Alcoholism relapse may provide advantages to families. AMERSA National Conference, Bethesda, MD.

Liepman, MR, Nirenberg, TD, Silvia, LY, Doolittle, RH, Begin, AM, & Broffman, TE. May (1990). Using the MFAD with alcoholic families. First International Conference on the McMaster Model, Providence, RI.

Liepman, MR, Silvia, LY, & Nirenberg, TD. (1989). The use of Family Behavior Loop Mapping for substance abuse. *Family Relations 38:*282-7.

Liepman, MR, Wolper, B, & Vazquez, J. (1982). An ecological approach for motivating women to accept treatment for chemical dependency. In BG Reed, J Mondanaro, GM Beschner. Eds. *Treatment Services for Drug Dependent Women*, Vol. II, Rockville, MD: NIDA, U.S. Government Printing Office, Publication #(ADM) 82-1219.

Linehan, MM. (1993). *Cognitive-Behavioral Treatment of Borderline Personality Disorder*. New York: Guilford.

Marlatt, GA, & Gordon, JR. (1985). Relapse Prevention: Maintenance Strategies in the Treatment of Addictive Behaviors. New York: Guilford.

Martin, RA, Velicer, WF, & Fava, JL. (1996). Latent transition analysis to the stages of change for smoking cessation. *Addict Behav 21:*67-80.

Miller, WR, Rollnick, S. (1991). Motivational Interviewing: Preparing People to Change Addictive Behavior. New York: Guilford.

Minuchin, S. (1974). *Families and Family Therapy*. Cambridge, MA: Harvard University Press.

Nirenberg, TD, Liepman, MR, Begin, AM, Doolittle, RH, & Broffman, TE. (1990). The sexual relationship of male alcoholics and their female partners during periods of drinking and abstinence. *J Studies on Alcohol 51,* 565-8.

O'Farrell, TJ, Hooley, J, Fals-Stewart, W, & Cutter, HSG. (1998). Expressed emotion and relapse in alcoholic patients. *Journal of Consulting and Clinical Psychology, 66:*744-52.

Prochaska, JO, & DiClemente, CC. (1986). Towards a comprehensive model of change. In WR Miller & N Heather Eds. *Treating Addictive Behaviors: Processes of Change*, pp 3-27. New York: Plenum.

Silvia, LY, & Liepman, MR. (1991a). Family behavior loop mapping enhances treatment of alcoholism. *Family & Community Health 13,* 72-83.

Silvia, LY, & Liepman, MR: Hiding in a bottle: Family Behavior Loop Mapping (videotape). (1991b). Winston-Salem, NC, Bowman Gray School of Medicine [Contact Dr. Liepman].

Smilkstein, G. (1980). The cycle of family function: A conceptual model for family medicine. *Journal of Family Practice 11:*223-32.

Stanton, MD, & Shadish, WR. (1997). Outcome, attrition, and family-couples treatment for drug abuse: A meta-analysis and review of the controlled, comparative studies. *Psychological Bulletin 122:*170-91.

Steinglass, P, Davis, DI, & Berenson, D. (1977). Observations of conjointly hospitalized "alcoholic couples" during sobriety and intoxication: Implications for theory and therapy. *Family Process 16:*1-16.

Stevenson, RL. (1886). *Strange Case of Dr. Jekyll and Mr. Hyde*. London: Longmans & Green.

Wegscheider-Cruse, S. (1989). Another Chance: Hope and help for the alcoholic family. 2nd edition. Palo Alto, CA: Science & Behavior Books.

doi:10.1300/J020v26n01_04

EVIDENCE-BASED MODELS

Brief Strategic Family Therapy: Engagement and Treatment

Ervin Briones, PhD
Michael S. Robbins, PhD
José Szapocznik, PhD

SUMMARY. An overview of Brief Strategic Family Therapy (BSFT), a family-based, empirically validated intervention designed to treat children and adolescents' problem behaviors is presented. In this article

Ervin Briones is affiliated with the Department of Psychology at The University of Tennessee at Martin.

Michael S. Robbins and José Szapocznik are affiliated with the University of Miami.

Address correspondence to: Ervin Briones, Department of Psychology, The University of Tennessee at Martin, 329 Humanities, Martin, TN 38238 (E-mail: EBriones@utm.edu.) Inquiries on the approaches presented here should be sent to José Szapocznik (E-mail: jszapocz@med.miami.edu.)

This work was supported by a National Institute on Drug Abuse grant (CTNU10 DA 13720) to José Szapocznik, Principal Investigator.

[Haworth co-indexing entry note]: "Brief Strategic Family Therapy: Engagement and Treatment." Briones, Ervin, Michael S. Robbins, and José Szapocznik. Co-published simultaneously in *Alcoholism Treatment Quarterly* (The Haworth Press) Vol. 26, No. 1/2, 2008, pp. 81-103; and: *Family Intervention in Substance Abuse: Current Best Practices* (ed: Oliver J. Morgan, and Cheryl H. Litzke) The Haworth Press, 2008, pp. 81-103. Single or multiple copies of this article are available for a fee from The Haworth Document Delivery Service [1-800-HAWORTH, 9:00 a.m. - 5:00 p.m. (EST). E-mail address: docdelivery@haworthpress.com].

Available online at http://atq.haworthpress.com
© 2008 by The Haworth Press. All rights reserved.
doi:10.1300/J020v26n01_05

the theoretical underpinnings of BSFT are described using a clinical case to illustrate the basic BSFT tenets. A selected review of outcome evidence is presented as well as the considerable clinical development and research evidence on specialized BSFT Engagement. Clinical implementation is highlighted. doi:10.1300/J020v26n01_05 *[Article copies available for a fee from The Haworth Document Delivery Service: 1-800-HAWORTH. E-mail address: <docdelivery@haworthpress.com> Website: <http://www.HaworthPress.com>* © *2008 by The Haworth Press. All rights reserved.]*

KEYWORDS. Family therapy, adolescent, alcohol-other drug abuse, engagement, strategic, structural

INTRODUCTION

The Espinozas, headed by a single Venezuelan-born mother in her mid thirties, includes four offspring: 21 year old son serving time in prison, 19 year old daughter working full-time, a 14 year old son, Michael, currently on probation for burglary charges, and 16 year old, Juan, who was referred to treatment following a recent arrest. Juan is referred to by mother as "a cocaine baby"(i.e., she was using cocaine when Juan was in utero). At intake, Juan tested positive for marijuana, reported that he had dropped out of school and did not have a job. His mother reported that Juan did not help at home and spent the majority of his time with delinquent friends who used alcohol and other drugs and had problems at home. Ms. Espinoza reports that on two separate occasions she lost custody of her children due to her own drug use problems in the past. She reports being sober for 4 years and gainfully employed. Mother and children do not have a close relationship. In addition, mother is not successful in her attempts to manage her younger boys. Her parenting typically involves nagging her children, setting unrealistic goals, and sermonizing. The younger boys, particularly Juan, tend to withdraw when mother lectures. There is a lack of a positive affective relationship between mother and her younger boys. The younger boys are highly involved with each other, supporting each other's deviant behavior, including encouraging one another to disobey mother and court. Younger boys do not see that they have a problem and are reluctant to participate in treatment.

TARGET POPULATION

The example of the Espinoza family illustrates typical problems targeted by Brief Strategic Family Therapy (BSFT) and reflects the fact that BSFT was designed not only to treat adolescent drug use but also other behavioral problems that often accompany drug use (Jessor & Jessor, 1977; McGee & Newcomb, 1992), including lack of school bonding and underachievement, oppositional defiance, aggression, delinquency, sexually risky behavior, and disengagement from pro-social activities. Although the focus of BSFT is to address drug use and related behavior problems, therapists do this by working relationally with the entire family. That is, family relationships are targeted for change rather than individual problems. Specifically, BSFT addresses maladaptive patterns of interactions in the Espinoza family that are supporting the two younger boys' acting out behaviors within and outside the family. The initial treatment plan for the Espinoza family included several specific family goals: (1) decreasing anger and blaming toward the boys and in particular toward Juan, (2) restoring emotional connection between mother and children, (3) increasing mother's nurturance, (4) improving family members' ability to effectively negotiate and resolve differences of opinion, (5) elevating mother's hierarchy in the family (including helping her to be more effective in her parental management skills), and (6) establishing appropriate emotional boundaries between younger brothers. By impacting these aspects of family functioning, the two younger boys' behavior problems will decrease over the course of treatment if not disappear all together.

BRIEF STRATEGIC FAMILY THERAPY

Brief Strategic Family Therapy (BSFT) is a family-based, empirically validated intervention designed to treat children's and adolescents' problem behaviors. BSFT has evolved from more than thirty years of research and practice at the University of Miami Center for Family Studies. BSFT is an integrative approach dating back to the late 1970s, drawing on structural theory and techniques of Salvador Minuchin (e.g., Minuchin & Fishman, 1981), and the strategic thinking of Haley (1976) and Madanes (1981). In this article we describe: (a) the theoretical underpinnings of BSFT; (b) some of the evidence on BSFT; (c) the considerable clinical development and corresponding research on specialized BSFT Engagement techniques; and (d) the clinical implementation of BSFT.

The abbreviated BSFT manual for clinicians (Szapocznik, Hervis, & Schwartz, 2003) is available in hard copy, free of charge, from the National Institute on Drug Abuse (Ms. Gerry Murphy, Supervisor, National Clearinghouse for Alcohol & Drug Info, P.O. Box 2345, Rockville, Maryland 20847), or may be downloaded at http://www.drugabuse.gov/TXManuals/bsft/bsftindex.html.

Basic Assumptions

BSFT is based on the fundamental assumption that the family is the most proximal and influential context for child development (Szapocznik & Coatsworth, 1999). We view the family as the primary force shaping the way a child thinks, feels and behaves. Research demonstrates that family relations are predictors of drug abuse and related antisocial behaviors (cf. Szapocznik & Coatsworth, 1999). Research also shows, however, that adolescent drug abuse and behavior problems can change as a result of changes in family relations (Liddle & Dakof, 1995; Robbins, Alexander, & Turner, 2000). Family relations are thus believed to play a pivotal role in the evolution and/or maintenance of behavior problems including drug abuse, and consequently are a primary target for intervention.

BSFT recognizes that although the family is the primary context of human growth and development, the family itself is also part of a larger social system and–like a child is influenced by her/his family–the family is influenced by the larger social system in which it exists (Bronfenbrenner, 1979). This sensitivity to contextual or ecological factors begins with an understanding of the important influence of family but extends also to peers, school, and the neighborhood in creating protection or risk for behavior problems including drug abuse. BSFT also targets parents' relationships to their children's peers and schools, as well as the unique relationships that parents have with individuals (e.g., extended family members) and systems (e.g., work, support group) outside of the nuclear family. Hence, the target of BSFT is the family broadly defined to include the individuals who function in roles that are traditionally or legally assigned to family members.

Theoretical Underpinnings

BSFT is best articulated around three central constructs: system, structure/patterns of interactions, and strategy (Szapocznik & Kurtines, 1989).

System

The first construct is a systems approach. A system is an organized whole that is comprised of parts that are interdependent or interrelated. A family is a system that is comprised of individuals whose behaviors affect each other. Family members become accustomed to the behavior of other family members, because such behaviors have occurred thousands of times over many years. In the Espinoza family, one pattern that emerged over time involved the older sister taking on parental responsibilities for her younger brothers when the mother was separated from her children. Consequently, sister had developed a strong leadership position in the family that made it difficult for mother to gain a leadership role when she returned to the family. Also, because younger brothers were close in age and the older brother was immersed in deviant behaviors outside the home and was not physically or emotionally available, a special bond between younger siblings had taken place. These behaviors synergistically work together to organize the Espinoza family system.

Structure

The second construct is structure. A central characteristic of a system is that it is comprised of parts that interact with each other. The set of repetitive patterns of interactions that characterize a family is called the family's structure. A maladaptive family structure is characterized by repetitive family interactions such that family members repeatedly elicit the same unsatisfactory responses from other family members. In our example, as mother scolded Juan for misbehaving, Juan withdrew from mother and recruited his brother's support.

Strategy

The third fundamental concept of BSFT is strategy and is defined by interventions that are practical, problem-focused, and deliberate. Practical interventions are selected for their likelihood to move the family toward desired objectives. One important aspect of practical interventions is choosing to emphasize one aspect of a family's reality (e.g., mother nags because she cares for Juan's well-being) as a way to foster a parent-child connection, or another aspect (e.g., "this youth could get into serious problems at any moment") in another family with passive or permissive parents to heighten their sense of urgency and encourage their involvement and setting rules and consequences quickly. Either strategy will be used depending on how the family is responding to a youth's problem.

As a problem-focused approach, BSFT targets family interaction patterns that are directly relevant to the youth's symptoms. For example, Ms. Espinoza's ineffective parenting approach (nagging) and Juan's typical withdrawing response is a pattern directly related to mother's reliance on this way of connecting with her son. Interventions simultaneously attempt to appropriately connect mother and her children by strategically highlighting positive aspects of their relationship, facilitating parental nurturance, and helping Ms. Espinoza and her children effectively to negotiate rules and consequences.

Our intervention strategies are very deliberate, meaning that the therapist determines the maladaptive interactions that, if changed, are most likely to lead to our desired outcomes (i.e., adolescent prosocial behavior) in a planned fashion. For instance, before working on mother's behavior management, one has to work on reestablishing positive emotional connection between mother and children so mother's attempt to manage children's behavior can be accepted as mother's expression of concern and love for them and thus less likely to be resisted.

RESEARCH ON BSFT: TREATMENT AND ENGAGEMENT

Rather than review all research on BSFT, because of space limitations, only one study on BSFT treatment efficacy and one on BSFT engagement efficacy are reviewed.

Treatment Outcome

The efficacy of BSFT has been established in several studies. For example, a clinical trial randomized 126 Hispanic families with a behavior problem adolescent to one of two conditions: BSFT or Group Treatment Control (Santisteban, Coatsworth et al., 2003). At intake 52% of participant adolescents reported use of either alcohol or other drugs during the past month and 94% scored in the clinical range on one or both of two behavior problem scales (conduct disorder and socialized aggression) from the Revised Behavior Problem Checklist (RBPC; Quay & Peterson, 1987).

Compared to Group Treatment, BSFT cases showed significantly greater pre to post-intervention improvement in parent reports of adolescent conduct problems and antisocial behavior in the company of peers, adolescent reports of marijuana use, and observer ratings and self reports of family functioning. More specifically, there was a 75% clinical reduction on marijuana use, 58% reduction in association with antisocial peers, and 42% improvement in acting-out behavioral problems in the BSFT condition, all of which were significantly greater than the group treatment (cf. Santisteban et al., 2003).

Engagement Outcome

Engaging and retaining families of drug using and problem behavior adolescents is one of the most difficult challenges faced by therapists. For example, only 27.1% of drug using adolescents stay in outpatient community treatments for the minimum expected time (Hser et al., 2001). In a study with drug using, delinquent adolescents it was noted that in an unmodified "usual services condition," only 22% of the families received any substance abuse or mental health services (Henggeler, Pickrel, Brondino, & Crouch, 1996). These findings are particularly alarming because youth who drop out of treatment fare worse than treatment completers on measures of individual, school, home, and community functioning (Kazdin, Mazurick, & Seigel, 1994; Liddle & Dakof, 1995). In response to this problem, we developed a set of procedures based on BSFT principles to more effectively engage behavior problem, substance using youths and their families in treatment. This approach, which we call BSFT Engagement (Szapocznik & Kurtines, 1989), is based on the premise that resistance to entering treatment can be understood in family interactional terms.

The effectiveness of BSFT engagement has been established in several investigations. For example, a randomized clinical trial of BSFT Engagement vs. Engagement as Usual with drug using Hispanic adolescents and their families, demonstrated that 93% of families that received the BSFT Engagement were successfully engaged into treatment, compared to 42% of families that received Engagement as Usual (Szapocznik, Perez-Vidal et al., 1988). Moreover, the utilization of the same techniques to retain cases in treatment resulted in 77% of families in the BSFT Engagement condition receiving a full dose of therapy (approximately 8 sessions), compared to 25% of families in Engagement as Usual. Moreover, all families retained in both conditions (three times as many with BSFT Engagement than Engagement as Usual) showed significant improvements in drug use, conduct problems and family functioning. Although BSFT Engagement brought into treatment more difficult to engage families, once in treatment they benefited from

BSFT treatment like any other family (see also Coatsworth et al., 2001; Santisteban et al., 1996).

CLINICAL APPLICATION OF BSFT

In the following section we present the goals and main themes of BSFT using clinical examples; who is seen and in what format; and sequence of BSFT therapeutic techniques.

Goals and Main Themes of the Treatment Program

BSFT targets primarily changes in family interactions. Table 1 lists the specific change goals targeted in BSFT. Change goals for the Espinoza family included (1) decreasing anger and blaming toward the boys, (2) restoring positive emotional connection between mother and children, (3) increasing mother's nurturance, (4) improving family

TABLE 1. Change Goals of BSFT

Structural Level	Specific Goals
Family	Increased parental figures involvement with one another and improve the balance of involvement of the parent figures with the child
	Improved effective parenting, including successful management of children's behavior
	Improved family cohesiveness, collaboration, and affect, and reduced family negativity
	Improved "appropriate" bonding between children and parents
	Improved family communication, conflict resolution and problem solving skills
	Correct assignment and effective performance of the roles and responsibilities of the family
Individual child/adolescent	Reduced behavior problems
	Reduced substance use
	Bonding to family
	Improved self-control
	Development of prosocial behaviors
	Reduced associations with antisocial peers
	Good school attendance, conduct and achievement

members' ability to deal with conflict, (5) elevating mother's hierarchy in the family (including helping her to be more effective in her parental management skills), and (6) establishing appropriate emotional boundaries between younger brothers.

Who Is Seen and in What Format

BSFT involves the whole family in treatment. Services can be provided in the office or at the family's home. BSFT sessions typically take place once per week for approximately 8-16 weeks depending on the level of severity of the adolescent's problems and the number of family members presenting with symptoms (e.g., depressed mother, alcoholic father). Sessions can occur more frequently and this often happens, particularly around crisis times because these are opportune moments for change. Sessions typically run 1 to 1.5 hours. BSFT can be implemented in a variety of settings, including community social services agencies, mental health clinics, health agencies and family clinics. The Espinoza family, for instance, was seen 18 times in total including at the office, primarily in their home, and a few sessions in a residential treatment facility where Michael, youngest son, was sent as result of his second arrest. A very strong, positive emotional exchange took place between mother and Juan during the sixth session soon after Michael's second arrest.

Sequence of Therapy

BSFT is delivered as an integrated strategy that follows five sequential steps: (a) Joining, (b) Enactment, (c) Interactional Diagnosis, (d) Treatment Plan, and (e) Restructuring Change (see Figure 1). Each of these steps is crucial for effective change to occur. Without any of them, therapy with problem behavior adolescents often fails.

(a) Joining or Establishing a Therapeutic Relationship

Joining involves showing acceptance and respect for each family member and making them feel understood. The purpose of joining is to blend with the system to have the family accept the therapist as their leader as well as a member of the new "therapeutic system" that includes family and therapist. Joining strategies include mimicking the family style, validating or supporting family members, formulating personally

FIGURE 1. BSFT Change Sequence

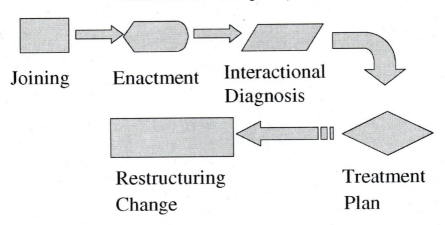

Joining   Enactment   Interactional
Diagnosis

Restructuring   Treatment
Change   Plan

meaningful goals, and attending to each client's experience (Diamond, Hogue, Liddle, & Dakof, 1999).

Accepting the family as they are during the initial phase of therapy and not challenging their maladaptive patterns is a strategic intervention given that families will be challenged to relate to one another differently later on, but only after they think we are on their "side." For instance, at the beginning of the first session with the Espinoza family, the older sister emphatically interrupted mother, "let's not talk about that," referring to the times when they were separated from mother. The therapist did not challenge the system but validated the family by saying, "I can see that this is a tough issue for both of you and your brothers to talk about." In the initial session, the therapist also observed that mother would persistently complain about Juan's behavior but would not give Juan a chance to respond. After reflecting back what the mother was saying without challenging her communication and parenting skills, the therapist validated Juan by saying "it must not be easy for you to hear your mom saying all those things at this moment. I wonder what you were thinking or feeling when she was saying all that to you." Juan shrugged but did not respond verbally. When asked specifically to respond to mother's statements, Juan replied emphatically: "I don't want to talk and I don't want to be here." The therapist, validating Juan, adds: "I don't blame you. I bet there must be a lot of other places that you would rather be right now. I appreciate your being up front with me about that. I am just pleased that you were able to be here today." Right after this, mother continued to sermonize Juan and lecture him about the importance of talking in therapy, finishing high school, and having a full time job. By rolling with the resistance, the therapist did not challenge any family member or the family organization.

The first step in BSFT then is to establish a therapeutic alliance with each family member and with the family as a whole. Challenging how the family functions prematurely, particularly challenging a powerful member in the family, can damage the therapeutic relationship with negative consequences such as one member's or the whole family's dropout, resistance to change, challenge to therapist's leadership, and lack of involvement in the therapeutic process. Indeed, research has shown that failure to maintain a balanced alliance with all family members can lead to early treatment dropout (Robbins et al., 2006).

(b) Creating Enactments

During the joining phase we create a therapeutic context where family members are free to interact in their typical style. By simply following family members' statements and non-verbal behaviors with questions (tracking) about how the family relates and reacts, sometimes families start interacting with one another as if the therapist was not present. These are called "spontaneous" enactments. Enactments permit the therapist to directly observe how the family behaves at home (outside of the session) and are critical for accurately identifying the family's characteristic pattern of interaction to properly assess family's strengths and diagnose maladaptive interactions that will guide the development of the treatment plan. It is the process of how the family interacts in the "here and now" that will be crucial in observing and diagnosing the interactional patterns. Therefore, BSFT is not interested in why problems got started. It is concerned with present observable interactions that, although they might have been the result of events that happened in the past, are alive today in the way family members relate to one another. For the Espinoza family, an enactment allowed us to observe: (1) the mother sermonize-Juan withdraw pattern of interaction, (2) daughter's powerful position in the family, and (3) the ineffective parenting behaviors.

(c) Interactional Diagnosis

It is necessary to know which interactions to strengthen and which to change. Such a determination is derived from BSFT diagnostic categories that organize all of the observations of a family's interactional patterns revealed during enactments. This diagnosis is critical for accurately identifying the family's characteristic patterns of interaction, i.e., the family's structure. BSFT diagnosis is comprised of five interrelated dimensions (Robbins, Hervis et al., 2001): (a) "Structure" measures leadership, subsystem organization, and communication flow; (b) "Resonance" measures the sensitivity of family members toward one another (focusing on boundaries and emotional distance between family members); (c) "Developmental Stage" measures the extent to which each family member's roles and tasks are consistent with what would be expected, given his or her age and family role; (d) "Identified Patienthood" measures the extent to which family members view the symptom bearer (e.g., adolescent drug abuser) as the cause of all of the family's problems; and (e) "Conflict Resolution" identifies the family's style at addressing disagreements through denial, avoidance, diffusion or expression and negotiation of differences of opinion.

The BSFT Diagnosis is fully focused on what family members do (process), not on what they say (content). It helps to organize observed behavior into patterns of interactions; strategically identifies the interactional patterns that are most amenable to change or which represent the best points of entry; formulates specific and focused treatment plans to change maladaptive patterns of interactions. Emphasis is given to those family's problematic relations that are linked to the youth's problem behaviors, or that interfere with the parent's (or parent figure's) ability to correct the youth's problem behaviors. In our example, Ms. Espinoza does not communicate clearly with Juan about what she expects nor does she express her love and concern for him, rather she nags. She also becomes angry when trying to correct children's behaviors without following through with clear rules and consistent and fair consequences. Mother and daughter do not communicate clearly about parental leadership in the family, and thus they act as parents who compete and undermine each other.

(d) Treatment Plan

The main goal of the treatment plan is to guide the therapist in targeting change of the maladaptive interactional patterns that are identified during the diagnostic process to maximize efficiency and effectiveness. What will be changed is often evident from what has been observed. The therapist plans how s/he will intervene to help the family move from its present ways of interacting and the undesirable symptoms they produce, to more adaptive and successful ways of interacting that will eliminate these symptoms. Table 2 represents maladaptive patterns of interaction observed in families with adolescents who use drugs and have related behavior problems. Changing these maladaptive patterns into more successful ways of interacting will be an intrinsic part of the treatment plan.

(e) Restructuring or Change Producing Intervention

The interventions used to help families move from their maladaptive patterns of interactions to healthier ones are called restructuring. The restructuring phase in BSFT includes 5 sequential techniques: (1) highlighting; (2) reframing; (3) assigning task; (4) guiding or coaching; and (5) providing positive feedback.

TABLE 2. Maladaptive Patterns of Interaction Observed in Families with Adolescent Behavior Problems

Organization:
- Powerlessness in parent figures.
- Unbalance in the parental or executive subsystem.
- Powerful adolescents (drug user).
- Ineffective parenting.
- Disrespect of parents.
- Triangulated interactional sequences.
- Coalitions between one parental figure and the identified patient against all other parental figure(s).
- Lack of participation of the identified patient (drug user) in the sibling subsystem.

Resonance:
- User (Identified patient) and his/her "protector" are enmeshed.
- "Other" parent is distant, disengaged from both the user (adolescent) and the "protecting" parent.
- Close and enmeshed relationships are often very conflictive, but not truly intimate. Lots of arguments.

Conflict-Resolution:
- High levels of conflict, a pattern of non-resolution.
- Inability for constructive confrontation and negotiation.

Identified Patienthood:
- The "drug user" or "identified patient" is very centralized by virtue of high levels of negativity or being a constant topic of conversation.
- Identified patient is viewed as the source of most of the family pain and unhappiness.

Developmental Stage:
- The user is infantilized in that s/he functions at a lower level of roles and responsibilities within the home than expected for his/her age.
- Other siblings "pick up the slack" or "compensate for the family" by assuming roles and responsibilities beyond their age.

(1) Highlighting. After deciding which aspect of the present interaction will be restructured, the BSFT therapist "highlights" it. Highlight means to intensify or bring attention to an interactional pattern with the purpose of making explicit to the family what you just observed. Highlighting signals to the family that this is a place to stop, look, and listen. Highlights can be used to magnify either adaptive or maladaptive family transactions. A positive highlight is used to bring attention to an adaptive interaction with the purpose of capitalizing on the family's strengths. For instance, when Ms. Espinoza says in a low voice, "How much I want them to avoid my mistakes" and then goes into blaming, the BSFT therapist stops all conversation, turns to Juan and in a soft, warm voice says, "Did you hear what your mother just said? This is VERY important." During a session soon after the second arrest of Michael, Juan was visibly shaken by the possibility that his younger brother was going to be sent away to a more intense rehabilitation center or correctional facility. The therapist highlighted Juan's non-verbal behavior by saying: "It seems like you are very *worried* about your brother's future, *worried* about what this will mean to your family and *worried* about how it will impact your own relationship with your brother." Soon after this highlight Juan started softly sobbing.

A highlight can also be used to focus on a maladaptive interaction that needs to be changed. For example, after it was observed how Ms. Espinoza has been nagging Juan without engaging him in a conversation about how he feels about his brother being in jail, the therapist could say: "When you spoke with Juan about the impact that Michael's problems with the law has on your relationship with Juan, your son withdrew and you could not find out what he is thinking or feeling." This highlight could be used to bring into focus that Juan's withdrawal followed mother's attempt to speak with him. This can also be very effective in pointing out how certain behaviors work against the mom's personal goals of reconnecting with her sons in a positive way. Because highlighting maladaptive interactional patterns can be interpreted as an open attack against a particular family member or the whole system, it is essential that therapists include many joining statements, avoid confrontations or overtly challenge family members, and try to immediately provide an alternative view that supports a more positive interactional climate and that is more conducive for change as described in the next section.

(2) Reframing. Reframing is the formulation of a "different" perspective or "frame" of reality than the one within which the family has been operating. The therapist presents this new frame in a manner that

"sells" to the family the new frame in order to elicit a new way of interacting that is more adaptive. Examples of reframes with the Espinoza family are: "There is no doubt that you love your son. I can see that every time you begin to speak." "You have so much invested in him and you are terrified that something bad might happen to him. I can hear it in your tone of voice. You almost sound panicked to find something that is going to help him avoid his problems with drugs and the law." "Did you realize how much your son also feels for you? Every time you get upset, he shows how much he respects you by withdrawing to avoid disagreeing with you." "I can see how much you two love each other and want to make this work." Another reframe used when Juan started sobbing right after therapist highlighted how worried he was about his brother's future was, "You really care about your brother, you cry because you love your brother." To the mom, the therapist said: "He is a good kid. He is a very sensitive and caring young man."

It is important to note that in BSFT the goal of reframing is NOT to change individual cognition. Rather, the goal is to create a new context in which family interactions can occur. Reframing is often used to disrupt negative perceptions by offering positive alternatives to the family. Only by consistently attending to the love for each other that resulted from Ms. Espinoza's frustration and Juan's withdrawal will the therapist be able to induce more positive affect and alter the characteristic pattern of interactions through the assignment of therapeutic tasks.

(3) Assigning Therapeutic Task. Therapeutic tasks are specific actions that need to take place in session to achieve adaptive interactions. In fact, the therapeutic task assigned immediately after a reframe of a negative interactional pattern is intended to reverse the maladaptive interaction observed during the enactment phase. In the Espinoza family, instead of mother scolding the silent and angry son, the task is for the mother to express her pain and love for him and to pause to allow Juan to speak and express his thoughts or feelings (to increase proper communication and emotional connection). Instead of Ms. Espinoza nagging Juan about how he "could end up in the same situation" as his brother unless he changes, the task is to ask mom to comfort her son who is in deep pain for his brother (to increase nurturance). Instead of sermonizing, the task is for Ms. Espinoza to come up with clear rules and consequences about children's curfew and involve the adolescents in the process of negotiating fair consequences (to increase proper behavior management and elevate mother's hierarchical position in the family). In other words, the therapeutic tasks will be dictated by the interactional diagnosis derived from the enactments.

Because emphasis is in promoting new skills among family members, both at the level of individual behaviors and family interactions, tasks are the vehicle through which therapists compose opportunities for the family to behave differently. It is a general rule that the BSFT therapist must first assign a task to be performed within the session, where the therapist has an opportunity to observe, assist, and facilitate the successful completion of the task.

(4) Guiding or Coaching. Guiding involves leading the family, sometimes step by step, to interact in adaptive ways. Coaching involves modeling certain behaviors, teaching specific skills, or practicing with the family or a family member new ways of interacting. After highlighting an interactional pattern (technique 1), reframing (technique 2), and assigning a therapeutic task (technique 3), families often go back to old maladaptive patterns of relating because they are uncomfortable with the assigned task (i.e., "tell your son how much you love him," "reach out to your son and comfort him the best way you can now that he is crying," "tell your mom what feelings you have for your brother"), or simply do not have the skills to complete it well (i.e., "I don't know how to put into words what I'm feeling right now . . . I don't speak that way").

It is during this phase that the most intensive work for both the therapists and the families take place. For therapists, this phase includes guiding families to remain on task by blocking diffusions onto other topics ("that's an important topic to be addressed later but please let's go back to what you were doing before"), reversing negativity by the use of reframes ("I know you love your son so much that you want him to do many things at once but let's focus on one thing at a time"), assigning emotionally deeper tasks ("right now I would like you to look straight at your mother's eyes and tell her what those beautiful words mean to you"), and highlighting positive exchanges to extend the moment as much as possible ("What you just said so softly is very powerful and deserves to be heard again. Tell your mom what it means to you now that she is sober . . . say it with more passion . . . let her know your feelings," "Mom, tell your son how it feels to hear that your son is proud of you for being sober for 4 years," "Give your son a hug and hold him for a moment and pretend that he's not this tough 16 year old but that he is a boy who needs your comfort because he is hurting for his brother.").

(5) Positive Feedback. During and at the end of a successful transaction therapists should provide the family with positive feedback about what they did in the session as a way to highlight and reinforce healthy family interactions. This feedback has to be given in very concrete behavioral terms and should always be delivered to increase a sense of

competency in family members as well as to increase the likelihood that these new behaviors will occur again. With the Espinoza family, for instance, after mother had nurtured Juan by having listened to him attentively and touched him tenderly and held him in her arms while Juan cried for his brother, a BSFT therapist can add: "You guys did fantastic right now. Juan, it takes a brave young man to show how he really feels." "You did such a nice job comforting your son in such a tender way." "You listened and supported him." "Without your support, Juan may not have been able to express his thoughts and feelings about his brother."

Termination of Treatment

Termination occurs when it is clear that the family has met the goals of the treatment plan; that is, family functioning has improved and adolescent behavior problems have been reduced or eliminated. Thus, termination is not determined by the number of sessions provided, but by the improvement in identified behavioral criteria. BSFT is designed to be delivered in 8-16 sessions. However, more or less may be provided depending upon the success of intervention strategies. After successful termination, families may experience new problems (e.g., relapse, increase in family conflict). In these circumstances, booster sessions can be provided.

BSFT ENGAGEMENT

The very same principles that apply to the understanding of family functioning and treatment also apply to engaging families or a family member who "resists" entering or staying in therapy. As such, the same techniques described above to treat the family once all members come to therapy (i.e., joining, tracking, assigning tasks, interactional diagnosis, reframing, guiding and coaching) are also used to engage and retain family members who are reluctant to participate in therapy (c.f., Szapocznik et al., 2003). Consistent with the relational focus of BSFT, resistance to treatment is defined in terms of the family's interactional patterns that preclude the family and/or its individual members from participating in treatment. Therefore, BSFT engagement techniques are applied to overcome these patterns and are not aimed to permanently change the family (which is done once the family enters treatment).

BSFT Engagement begins with the first phone call. During this first contact, therapists often only have access to one person, typically a parent (usually the adolescent's mother). Effectively negotiating this first contact sets the stage for the entire process of treatment. Therapists must be very empathic and warm; while, at the same time, pursuing their own therapeutic agenda. This initial contact is thus important to join with the caller, but almost exclusively around the topic of getting all family members into treatment. In joining the caller, the therapist must be cautious to avoid forming any alliance against other family members. For instance, in our clinical case, the therapist validated and reframed Ms. Espinoza after she complained about Juan's behavior by saying, "It seems that you are really concerned about your son's behavior. It shows also that you care deeply about him." This is a strategic move because it achieves joining with the caller but does not form any alliance against Juan. During the first call, the therapist should also gather information about (a) who needs to be included in the family sessions, and (b) barriers that may keep key family members from participating in treatment.

By listening for and tracking the caller's comments about family interactions, the therapist gains valuable information about potential interactional patterns that may interfere with engagement. Since it is not possible to observe any enactments when calling, we can nevertheless infer some interactional patterns by asking process-oriented questions guided by the BSFT diagnostic categories. For example, the therapist can ask Ms. Espinoza, "How will you ask Michael and Juan to come to treatment? What happens when you ask Michael to come? And, when he gets angry at you for asking him to come to treatment, what do you do next?" Based on the caller's responses to these key questions, it may be necessary for the therapist to speak directly with some or all family members over the phone prior to conducting the first session.

In general, the decision to contact additional family members is based on what the current patterns (as conveyed by the caller) suggest. If it is clear that the caller is not going to be effective in brining other family members into treatment, therapists must position themselves to create the bridge between other family members and treatment. That is, therapists must directly contact family members rather than rely on the caller. Common examples of when it is important to contact other family members are families in which a member is disengaged from other family members, or families in which the IP is the most powerful member in the family. In these two examples, it is essential for therapists to go directly to the disengaged family member or to the IP, respectively.

Another way to uncover the patterns for resistance to treatment is to assign exploratory tasks. After noticing that Ms. Espinoza justified Michael's potential absence, the therapist suggested to Ms. Espinoza that she ask Michael to come for her sake, not because there is anything wrong with him. Ms. Espinoza then says to the therapist, "I can't really ask him for my sake, because I know this is the only time when he goes out to play with his friends and it's just not fair . . . and also I know what he will say." By assigning this exploratory task, the therapist tracked that mother was protecting the system, by justifying Michael's absence, and identified that there was a strong emotional alliance between Juan and his younger brother. In light of these two patterns, the therapist validated mother by stating, "I can sense your frustration in wanting to get help and not getting any cooperation from Michael (validation). I see that you are a very sensitive mom who understands the need for adolescents to have friends and because you want harmony in the family so much, you don't even want to take the chance to upset your son" (reframe to join). Also, I've heard how important Michael is for you and how close Juan feels to his brother (validation) which tells me that Michael is a very important member in this family and we need his input in order to help the family. I know how important it is for you to have unity in your family and that you are not comfortable with confronting him, but I also noticed that you recognize how important he is in this family. May I help you in getting Michael to come to the sessions? Do I have your permission to call him myself?"

After getting permission and exploring the best ways to reach Michael, the therapist then begins the process of engaging him into treatment. During the first call with Michael, the therapist's goals were to join with him, find out how he views his family and therapy, and ultimately, implement reframes and assign tasks to engage him in family therapy. In doing so, the therapist said, "Michael, your mom and Juan speak so much about you in therapy. They really seem to value your opinion so much that it would be very important for your mom and especially for Juan if you were present when we have our sessions. I need your help because I've seen how important you are in your family, so without you I won't be able to help your family as much as you guys deserve. I promise I will not accuse you or make you do or say anything that you don't like. Your presence will be enough. Can I count on you being here tomorrow at 5:00 PM?" Michael was present in the next three sessions until he was arrested for the second time.

In circumstances in which the caller places a barrier to getting other family members involved in treatment, it is often necessary to validate the caller's concerns, highlight their commitment to the family, and reframe other family members' involvement in therapy. An effective reframing strategy involves helping the caller to see that getting other family members involved in treatment will help the caller meet their own personal goals for the family (e.g., reframing the importance of parents working effectively as a team will help mom in her goal to save her son).

Despite implementing intensive engagement strategies, it is not uncommon for one or more family members to fail to show up for the first session. Likewise, family members (and the entire family) may miss sessions over the course of treatment. Anytime there are missed sessions or the therapist believes that there is a chance a family (or family member) may miss a session, we expect therapists to adopt the aggressive engagement philosophy we have described. Thus, engagement and retention is an ongoing process. Therapists should be conducting a continuous evaluation to determine if the family is at risk for dropping out of treatment and implementing strategies to prevent failures to retain the family in treatment.

While the therapist makes some assumptions about the general direction in which a client/family should move from maladaptive behaviors to those that are personally and socially more adjusted, what is critically important is that the therapist does not challenge the system initially. As we take each step, we ask the relevant family members permission to take that step. A more in-depth coverage of BSFT engagement rationale and varied clinical examples are offered elsewhere (Szapocznik et al., 2003) in addition to one-person BSFT techniques and its empirical evidence (Szapocznik et al., 1983; 1986).

CONCLUSION

Throughout the mental health and drug abuse field, there is a substantial gap between the interventions, such as BSFT, validated in research studies and community practice (Institute of Medicine, 1998). In light of this gap, a major thrust of our current research efforts is to test the effectiveness of BSFT in community settings and to establish the mechanisms for training BSFT providers on a large scale. Currently, we are conducting a large, multi-site treatment study within the National Institute on Drug Abuse Clinical Trials Network (NIDA U10-DA13720). This study includes 480 drug using adolescents and their family members recruited from 8 community agencies from across the country, including a site in Puerto Rico. In this study, the effectiveness of BSFT is being compared to treatment as usual services at participating agencies.

To facilitate effectiveness trials and the dissemination of BSFT, the Center for Family Studies has established a Training Institute. One of the first products of the Training Institute was the completion of an updated version of the BSFT Manual (Szapocznik, Hervis, & Schwartz, 2003). The revised manual presents BSFT with the most recent clinical developments supported by efficacy findings, and was written specifically for clinicians in community treatment settings.

· The Training Institute trains therapists and clinical supervisors. Goals of the training program involve facilitating the appropriate implementation of BSFT in different settings (e.g., in-patient and out-patient clinics, community organizations, prevention programs) with diverse populations. Training is being offered locally, across the country and abroad. The training process has been standardized and includes taped family sessions that illustrate different aspects of the model, a didactic/interactive power point presentation, review of videotaped sessions with consented families, and review/supervision of active cases. The Training Institute is also in the process of developing procedures for credentialing therapists. For more information on BSFT training, see www.cfs.med.miami. edu/Docs/Training.htm.

REFERENCES

Bronfenbrenner, U. (1979). *The ecology of human development.* Cambridge, MA: Harvard University Press.

Coatsworth, J. D., Santisteban, D., McBride, C. K., & Szapocznik, J. (2001). Brief strategic family therapy versus community control: Engagement, retention, and an exploration of the moderating role of adolescent symptom severity. *Family Process, 40,* 313-332.

Diamond, G. M., Liddle, H. A., Hogue, A., & Dakof, G. A. (1999). Alliance-building interventions with adolescents in family therapy: A process study. *Psychotherapy: Theory, Research, Practice, Training, 36,* 355-368.

Grella, C. E., Joshi, V., & Hser, Y. I. (2004). Effects of comorbidity on treatment processes and outcomes among adolescents in drug treatment programs. *Journal of Child & Adolescent Substance Abuse, 13,* 13-31.

Haley, J. (1976). *Problem solving therapy.* San Francisco, CA: Jossey-Bass.

Henggeler, S. W., Pickrel, S. G., Brondino, M. J., & Crouch, J. L. (1996). Eliminating (almost) treatment dropout of substance abusing or dependent delinquents through home-based multisystemic therapy. *The American Journal of Psychiatry, 153,* 427-428.

Hser, Y. I., Grella, C. E., Hubbard, R. L., Hsieh, S. C., Fletcher, B. W., Brown, B. S. et al. (2001). An evaluation of drug treatments for adolescents in four United States cities. *Archives of General Psychiatry, 58,* 689-695.

Institute of Medicine. (1998). Bridging the gap between practice and research: Forging partnerships with community-based drug and alcohol treatment. Washington, DC, National Academy Press.

Jessor, R., & Jessor, S. L. (1977). *Problem behavior and psychosocial development: A longitudinal study of youth.* New York: Academic Press.

Kazdin, A. E., Mazurick, J. L., & Seigel, T. C. (1994). Treatment outcome among children with externalizing disorder who terminate prematurely versus those who complete psychotherapy. *Journal of the American Academy of Child and Adolescent Psychiatry, 33,* 549-557.

Liddle, H. A., & Dakof, G. A. (1995). Family based treatment for adolescent drug use: State of the science. Rahdert, E. 218-254. Rockville, MD. National Institute on Drug Abuse. Adolescent drug abuse: Clinical assessment and therapeutic interventions.

Madanes, C. (1981). *Strategic family therapy.* San Francisco: Jossey-Bass.

McGee, L., & Newcomb, M. D. (1992). General deviance syndrome: Expanded hierarchical evaluations at four ages from early adolescence to adulthood. *Journal of Consulting and Clinical Psychology, 60,* 766-776.

Minuchin, S., & Fishman, H. C. (1981). *Family therapy techniques.* Cambridge, MA: Harvard University Press.

Quay, H. G., & Peterson, D. R. (1987). Manual for the Revised Behavior Problem Checklist. University of Miami.

Robbins, M. S., Alexander, J. F., & Turner, C. W. (2000). Disrupting defensive family interactions in family therapy with delinquent adolescents. *Journal of Family Psychology, 14,* 688-701.

Robbins, M. S., Hervis, O. E., Mitrani, V. B., & Szapocznik, J. (2001). Assessing changes in family interaction: The Structural Family Systems Ratings. In P. K. Kerig & K. M. Lindahl (Eds.), *Family observational coding systems: Resources for systemic research* (pp. 207-224). Hillsdale, NJ: Erlbaum.

Robbins, M. S., Liddle, H. A., Turner, C. W., Dakof, G. A., Alexander, J. F., & Kogan, S. M. (2006). Adolescent and parent therapeutic alliances as predictors of dropout in multidimensional family therapy. *Journal of Family Psychology, 20,* 108-116.

Santisteban, D., Szapocznik, J., Perez-Vidal, A., Kurtines, W. M., Murray, E. J., & LaPerriere, A. (1996). Efficacy of intervention for engaging youth and families into treatment and some variables that may contribute to differential effectiveness. *Journal of Family Psychology, 10,* 44.

Santisteban, D., Coatsworth, J. D., Perez-Vidal, A., Kurtines, W. M., Schwartz, S., & LaPerriere, A. et al. (2003). Efficacy of Brief Strategic Family Therapy in modifying Hispanic adolescent behavior problems and substance use. *Journal of Family Psychology, 17,* 121-133.

Szapocznik, J., & Coatsworth, J. D. (1999). An ecodevelopmental framework for organizing the influences on drug abuse: A developmental model of risk and protection. In M.Glantz & C. R. Hartel (Eds.), *Drug Abuse: Origins and Interventions* (pp. 331-366). Washington, DC: American Psychological Association.

Szapocznik, J., Hervis, O. E., & Schwartz, S. (2003). *Brief Strategic Family Therapy for adolescent drug use* (Rep. No. 03-4751). Rockville, MD: National Institute on Drug Abuse.

Szapocznik, J., & Kurtines, W. M. (1989). *Breakthroughs in family therapy with drug abusing problem youth.* New York: Springer.

Szapocznik, J., Kurtines, W., Foote, F., Perez-Vidal, A., & Hervis, O. E. (1983). Conjoint versus one person family therapy: Some evidence for the effectiveness of conducting family therapy through one person. *Journal of Consulting and Clinical Psychology, 51,* 889-899.

Szapocznik, J., Kurtines, W., Foote, F. et al. (1986). Conjoint versus one person family therapy: Further evidence for the effectiveness of conducting family therapy through one person. *Journal of Consulting and Clinical Psychology, 54,* 395-397.

Szapocznik, J., Perez-Vidal, A., Brickman, A., Foote, F. H., Santisteban, D., Hervis, O. E. et al. (1988). Engaging adolescent drug abusers and their families into treatment: A strategic structural systems approach. *Journal of Consulting and Clinical Psychology, 56,* 552-557.

doi:10.1300/J020v26n01_05

Multidimensional Family Therapy
for Adolescent Alcohol Abusers

Cynthia L. Rowe, PhD
Howard A. Liddle, EdD

SUMMARY. Multidimensional Family Therapy (MDFT) has been empirically supported in a series of randomized clinical trials over 20 years. These studies have demonstrated the potency of MDFT in achieving outcomes across functional areas of the teen's life, including reductions in alcohol-other drug use, behavioral problems, emotional symptoms, negative peer associations, school failure, and deficits within the family. This article describes our approach to refining and testing MDFT with teens who abuse alcohol. Drawing from the research base on risk and protective factors for teen alcohol abuse and relapse patterns, a strong case can be made for using a family-based approach for adolescent alcohol problems. MDFT shows promising preliminary results with teens who have alcohol and marijuana use disorders. Specific change targets within

---

Cynthia L. Rowe is Investigator at The Center for Treatment Research on Adolescent Drug Abuse, which is part of the University of Miami Leonard M. Miller School of Medicine.

Howard A. Liddle is Principal Investigator and Director of the Center.

Address correspondence to: Howard A. Liddle, Center for Treatment Research on Adolescent Drug Abuse, P.O. Box 016069, Univ. of Miami School of Medicine, Miami, FL 33101-6069 (E-mail: h.liddle@miami.edu). The Center website location is: http://www.med.miami.edu/ctrada/#

[Haworth co-indexing entry note]: "Multidimensional Family Therapy for Adolescent Alcohol Abusers." Rowe, Cynthia L., and Howard A. Liddle. Co-published simultaneously in *Alcoholism Treatment Quarterly* (The Haworth Press) Vol. 26, No. 1/2, 2008, pp. 105-123; and: *Family Intervention in Substance Abuse: Current Best Practices* (ed: Oliver J. Morgan, and Cheryl H. Litzke) The Haworth Press, 2008, pp. 105-123. Single or multiple copies of this article are available for a fee from The Haworth Document Delivery Service [1-800-HAWORTH, 9:00 a.m. - 5:00 p.m. (EST). E-mail address: docdelivery@haworthpress.com].

this empirically supported family-based intervention for adolescent alcohol problems are outlined. doi:10.1300/J020v26n01_06. *[Article copies available for a fee from The Haworth Document Delivery Service: 1-800-HAWORTH. E-mail address: <docdelivery@haworthpress.com> Website: <http://www.HaworthPress.com> © 2008 by The Haworth Press. All rights reserved.]*

KEYWORDS. Alcohol abuse, adolescents, family therapy

INTRODUCTION

The last decade has seen significant advances in the empirical development and testing of treatments for adolescent alcohol abuse (Lowman, 2004). Individual and group interventions for adolescent alcohol problems are gaining empirical support, and researchers have made important discoveries outlining the critical factors and processes in alcohol relapse. Several studies have documented that standard community treatment can decrease adolescent alcohol use and ameliorate alcohol use disorders. However, in the first year following standard community-based treatment, up to 64% of teens continue, resume or increase their alcohol use (Maisto et al., 2001). Longer outcome studies show that over time (1-8 years), use of alcohol steadily rises in each consecutive year following standard, inpatient alcohol and drug treatment (Tapert et al., 2003). There is strong evidence that adolescents with alcohol use disorders are an underserved population at risk for chronic problems without effective treatment (Grant et al., 2006).

Risk and Protective Factors for Adolescent Alcohol Use Disorders

Alcohol problems are understood within a "biopsychosocial matrix of risk" (Zucker, 1994), which considers the multiple interacting influences that make individuals vulnerable for alcohol problems throughout the life span. Alcohol use in adolescence is generally embedded within a constellation of other deviant behaviors, including school failure, conduct problems, and drug use, which operate together to increase vulnerability for alcohol dependence in young adulthood and beyond (Guo et al., 2001). However, the risk factors for alcohol and other drug problems may be somewhat different (Zhou et al., 2006) and alcohol problems are known to have multiple interacting precipitating contributors, as well as different developmental trajectories. Generally, the earlier these problems develop and the greater the number of risk factors in the absence of protective factors, the poorer the prognosis for long-term development. Thus, contemporary research supports multi-component interventions for adolescent alcohol abuse that are developmentally oriented and capable of addressing these interrelated factors (IOM, 1990).

Family factors play a central role in early alcohol use and the progression of alcohol problems. A range of family risk factors have been consistently linked to adolescent alcohol problems, including parent and sibling substance use (Sher et al., 1991), poor parental monitoring (Kuperman, 1999), family conflict (Dishion & Medici-Skaggs, 2000), parents' alcohol norms (Brody et al., 2000), and low family support and control (Windle, 1996). Negative parenting behaviors not only predict initial levels of drinking, but also influence increases in drinking over time. Family factors are also among the strongest protective influences against adolescent alcohol problems. Longitudinal research suggests that firm parental rules against drinking at ages 10 and 16 reduce the likelihood of alcohol abuse and dependence at age 21 (Guo, 2001). Parental control also predicts de-escalation of drinking among high school teens who have initiated alcohol use (Stice et al., 1998). Even among high-risk families, protective factors still operate; young adolescents with alcoholic parents are protected from later alcohol problems through high levels of family organization and behavioral coping (Hussong & Chassin, 1997). A recent study suggests that the strength of the bond between the teen and parent may be more powerful in predicting teen drinking than family structure or parental drinking (Kuntsche & Kuendig, 2006).

Family factors also play an important mediational role in explaining the impact of other risk factors for problem drinking among adolescents. One of the most important protective functions of parents during adolescence is reducing the teen's association with drug using peers. Family risk factors predict the teen's migration toward drinking peers, which directly influences alcohol use (Blanton et al., 1997). Parent-child conflict also predicts increases in adolescents' and their friends' substance use over time. An 18-year longitudinal study uncovered strong direct effects of peer antisociality on adolescents' substance use, but showed that peer relationships were determined by a range of family factors in early childhood (Garnier & Stein, 2002). While peers exert direct effects on teen drinking, parents mediate these influences through several different mechanisms. Family factors appear to operate both directly and indirectly to contribute to teen drinking, indicating the need for effective family-based interventions.

Rationale for Family-Based Interventions for Adolescent Alcohol Abuse

A strong tradition exists for the use of family-based interventions for adult alcohol abusers (O'Farrell and Fals-Stewart, 2003). For instance, Behavioral Couples Therapy (BCT), recognized as one of the most promising interventions for alcoholism, helps alcoholics reduce their drinking and incidents of domestic violence with significant cost-savings up to 2 years post-treatment. By improving marital/couple interactions and reducing substance abuse, children's behavioral functioning also improves dramatically (Kelley and Fals-Stewart, 2002). Empirical support for both behavioral family therapy and family systems approaches in treating adult alcohol abusers has accumulated steadily (Stanton and Shadish, 1997). The success of these interventions serves as a solid platform for the application of family-based interventions for adolescent alcohol abusers.

Findings from several well-controlled clinical trials also support the comparative efficacy of family-based therapy in reducing levels of adolescent drug use and increasing adaptive functioning (Rowe and Liddle, 2003). Family-based interventions have been found to have superior pre–to post-treatment effects on levels of adolescent drug use compared to individual therapy, adolescent group therapy, and family psychoeducational counseling (Azrin et al., 1994; Henggeler et al., 1991; Liddle, 2002b; Liddle et al., 2001, 2004). These effects have been retained up to 12 months after termination (e.g., Liddle et al., 2001). Family-based interventions not only directly reduce drug use, but also consistently alter the multiple risk factors that predict progression into further dysfunction. However, these models have generally not been developed specifically with alcohol abusing samples, and few report effects on alcohol use.

There is some evidence that family-based interventions reduce alcohol use and related problems among teens. For instance, the Purdue Brief Family Therapy model significantly reduced adolescent alcohol use in fewer sessions than drug education and individually-oriented treatment as usual (Trepper et al., 1993). Azrin and colleagues demonstrated the superiority of behavioral family therapy in comparison to supportive counseling in reducing adolescent alcohol use and increasing the length of abstinence up to 9 months following treatment (Azrin et al., 1994). Further, family-based preventive interventions are among the most promising approaches for reducing the risk of alcohol abuse among adolescents. By reducing risk and bolstering protective factors, family-based interventions may be instrumental in reducing vulnerability for later alcohol problems. For instance, Project Northland, a multifaceted, multi-year community-based intervention with a strong family component, has been successful in reducing alcohol use among young adolescents, reducing peer risk and positive expectations about drinking, and improving parent-child communication relative to controls (Perry et al., 1996). Thus family-based interventions, which have the advantage of directly addressing the multiple interacting risk factors for alcohol abuse and bolstering protective mechanisms within the family and other systems, appear to hold promise in reducing teen drinking.

Multidimensional Family Therapy for Adolescent Substance Abuse

Multidimensional Family Therapy (Liddle, 2002a) is recognized as a "Best Practice" model for teen substance abuse and delinquency by federal and international agencies (Communities that Care, 2004; Drug Strategies, 2003; NIDA, 1999; CSAT, 1998; Rigter et al., 2004). It has demonstrated efficacy in several clinical trials over the past 20 years in reducing substance use and related problems, and in increasing the prosocial and protective functioning of teens and their families (Liddle, 2002b; Liddle et al., 2001; Liddle et al., 2004). There is also evidence of its potential as a prevention model to reverse adverse developmental trajectories among high-risk youth (Hogue et al., 2002). However, adolescents with primary alcohol use disorders have constituted only a small percentage of the samples studied in these clinical trials. Family-based models such as MDFT offer promise for treating alcohol abusing teens and their families (Lowman, 2004); however, more attention to the unique needs of alcohol abusing youth and their families is needed.

MDFT has been adapted for different clinical populations using a systematic, empirically-grounded treatment development framework. The model has evolved over the past 20 years in response to the unique clinical needs of different clinical populations, empirical advances in our understanding of the clinical phenomenon of adolescent substance abuse, and treatment outcome and process research findings that guide our clinical approach. Consistent with treatment development guidelines (Kazdin, 1994), the model has undergone rigorous tests of therapeutic process and outcome. Model developers have asked questions about the specific adolescent, parent, family, and environmental factors that influence treatment outcomes with each unique population. Specific intervention targets have been identified through careful examination of basic developmental and applied research, as well as exploration of key

MDFT processes linked to successful outcomes, and MDFT has been modified accordingly for unique populations. These different versions of the approach are designed to more effectively target the needs of different groups of adolescent substance abusers, such as adolescent girls, adolescents from different cultural backgrounds, and adolescents with multiple comorbid problems.

Previous studies have tested the impact of systematic variations of the MDFT model. For instance, in applying the model with young African-American urban male drug abusers, we explored the cultural themes being expressed in therapy, studied the literature on the risk and protective forces at work in the lives of urban African American teens, and adapted the approach to integrate this content (Jackson-Gilfort et al., 2001). More recently, a similar process has been undertaken to identify salient cultural themes that are critical for successful engagement and productive work with Hispanic youth and families. In another study, examination of alliance building interventions with adolescents who initially demonstrated poor therapeutic relationships enabled us to develop early stage interventions necessary to succeed in engaging teens in MDFT (Diamond et al., 2000). Similarly, this systematic empirically-driven treatment development approach has guided our efforts to refine the model for young adolescents (Rowe et al., 2003). These efforts have identified core mechanisms of change in family-based treatment, as well as helping to develop more effective methods of intervention for these specific groups and others.

Similar work has been done to adapt MDFT specifically for alcohol abusing teens. We have identified core areas based on etiological and treatment research that are potential targets of intervention. As we have done in previous treatment development efforts, we have worked from a detailed and deep understanding of the clinical phenomena of adolescent alcohol abuse, as we know it through the empirical literature, to identify areas of further development. The following sections describe this treatment development process and change targets within MDFT.

MULTIDIMENSIONAL FAMILY THERAPY
FOR ADOLESCENT ALCOHOL ABUSERS

The MDFT theory of change follows directly and logically from a multidimensional theory of dysfunction. Understanding that the teen's drinking and related problems have been caused by a complex set of interrelated and mutually reinforcing risk factors, MDFT targets change in each of these core areas of functioning. The model posits that reductions in target symptoms and increases in prosocial behaviors occur via multiple pathways, in differing contexts, and through different mechanisms. With the adolescent, the therapist seeks to transform the youth's substance using lifestyle into a developmentally normative one with improved functioning across domains, including promoting positive peer relations, healthy identity formation, bonding to school and other prosocial institutions, and autonomy within the parent-adolescent relationship. Goals with the parent include increasing parental commitment and preventing parental abdication, improving communication with the adolescent, and increasing knowledge and skills in the realm of parenting practices (e.g., limit-setting, monitoring). In family sessions, MDFT therapists aim to transform negative interactional patterns into more positive relationships and to promote supportive and effective communication among family members. The therapy is phasically organized, and it relies on success in one phase of the therapy before moving on to the next. Knowledge of normal development and developmental psychopathology guides the overall therapeutic strategy and specific interventions.

The format of MDFT has been modified to suit the clinical needs of different clinical populations. A full course of MDFT is delivered in several sessions each week over four to six months. Sessions may be held in a variety of contexts including in the home, clinic, other community settings (e.g., school), or by phone. The MDFT treatment system assesses and intervenes into four main areas: the adolescent as an individual, the parent/parents as a subsystem, the family interactional system, and the extrafamilial system (the family and adolescent's interactions and relationships with influential systems outside of the family). Assessment of functioning in each of these areas is followed by interventions into these same domains. The core interventions of MDFT are organized according to the particular subsystem targeted and the stage of treatment.

Treatment development efforts with MDFT have focused on addressing the risk factors specifically linked to teen alcohol problems and bolstering protective processes that have been shown to facilitate resiliency among teens at risk. These specific areas of focus are discussed below: alcohol expectancies, parental substance abuse, and family-based relapse prevention.

Alcohol Expectancies

Research has shown that adolescents' alcohol expectancies are a significant predictor of heavy and problem drinking (Colder and Chassin, 1999). Alcohol expectancies include beliefs about the positive social (e.g., appearing more comfortable) and emotional (e.g., feeling more relaxed) effects of alcohol, as well as beliefs that alcohol is less harmful and more normative than it actually is. Adolescents' alcohol expectancies and attitudes are closely linked to the norms families communicate about drinking and by parents' drinking patterns (Martino et al., 2006). Positive alcohol expectancies predict early initiation of alcohol use and determine progressive increases in alcohol use after initiation. Alcohol expectancies also predict relapse to alcohol use up to 8 years following treatment (Tapert et al., 2003).

Expectancies about the positive social effects of alcohol play an important role in adolescent alcohol problems but are explained at least partially by family factors. Alcohol expectancies are shaped not only by the teen's drinking experience, but also by parents' drinking. Children not only adopt their parents' drinking behaviors, but also the drinking coping strategies and motivations that are modeled by their parents (Windle, 1996). Children tend to internalize their parents' norms about drinking by early adolescence, and, once internalized, directly influence their drinking behaviors (Brody et al., 2000). Protective factors that are facilitated in healthy family environments, such as good decision making skills, self efficacy and positive coping, as well as social competence, reduce risk for adolescent alcohol problems. Clinical research shows that one prevention approach that intervened with parents (Project Northland) was successful in decreasing adolescents' positive alcohol expectancies (Perry et al., 1996).

MDFT attends to the social cognitive aspects of substance use, the meaning and motivation for substance use, the teen's developmental challenges, and motivation to improve one's life. Addressing expectancies, beliefs, and attitudes about alcohol is consistent with the MDFT therapist's work with the individual adolescent in that therapists challenge teens to examine their motivations for using and help them become aware of the health compromising aspects that are associated with substance use. Individual sessions with the adolescent focus on highlighting discrepancies between stated personal goals or outcomes and current lifestyle choices, including beliefs about substances. Continued use of substances is acknowledged as being incompatible with a non-substance using lifestyle and the benefits of this new lifestyle and the changes associated with it. Doing better in school, having less conflict at home, resolving one's legal problems, and having more fulfilling peer relations are elements of the non-substance using lifestyle that are developed and sought in MDFT.

The pathways to achieve a shift in alcohol expectancies and accompanying reductions in drinking come through individual work with the youth in ways that motivate him or her individually, but also in ways that involve parents and other systems. Work with the parents to examine their messages about alcohol use and norms about drinking are critical, in part because most parents underestimate their own teen's drinking (Guilamo-Ramos et al., 2006). The MDFT therapist helps parents in these individual sessions to commit to taking a firm stand against drinking and communicating a clear and consistent message that drinking is not safe for teens and is not acceptable. Individual work with both adolescents and parents provides a platform for families to talk together about drinking and other drug use. The therapist uses the core family therapy technique of enactment to shape productive and positive conversations between parents and teens that demonstrate the parents' love and concern for the adolescent in setting clear limits about drinking. These family sessions help the adolescent develop more realistic beliefs about alcohol and its consequences and hone new skills to avoid drinking.

Parental Alcoholism

One of the strongest and most consistent family risk factors for teen alcohol problems is parental alcoholism (Sher et al., 1991), with increased risk even when the parent's alcoholism is in remission. Lifetime risk of alcohol dependence is substantially elevated among children of alcoholics, particularly among those who initiate drinking during adolescence (Guo et al., 2001). Children with alcoholic parents show increased risk in the form of behavioral problems as young as age 3 (Fitzgerald et al., 1993), with high levels of drinking by either mother or father predicting heavy alcohol use as early as 5th and 6th grade (Weinberg et al., 1994). While genetics probably determines much of the liability for transition of alcoholism, environmental factors increase alcohol risk among children of alcoholics. Ellis et al. (1997) argue that it is the aggregation of numerous alcohol-specific (e.g., parental modeling) and alcohol-nonspecific factors (e.g., family disorganization) that increase risk for children of alcoholics. Parental alcoholism increases young adolescents' risk of alcohol abuse through specific mechanisms that can be addressed in family interventions, such as family conflict and lack of cohesion

(Havey & Dodd, 1995); decreased monitoring (Chassin et al., 1996); and behavior problems (Hussong et al., 1998). Parental alcohol use is an important determinant of alcohol-specific rules and alcohol availability in the home, which both predict teen drinking (Van Zundert et al., 2006). Thus, the genetic transmission of alcohol problems from parent to child is most likely mediated in part by factors that can be altered through intervention (Sher, 1994).

Directly and systematically addressing parental alcoholism is consistent with core parent work in MDFT. MDFT targets the functioning of the parent as an individual adult, apart from his or her role as a parent or caregiver. Since parenting practices are correlated with functioning in other domains of a parent's life, these other aspects of a parent's day-to-day functioning (e.g., mental health issues, drug or alcohol abuse, marital disharmony) are germane to address in therapy. The therapist motivates parents to take steps to change their own lives by resuscitating their love and commitment for the child, and by highlighting the links between the parent's own functioning, their parenting deficits, and the child's problems. The therapist helps parents see how their drinking and other substance use has impacted the teen and how the parents' recovery is a necessary part of the youth's ability to get sober and stay abstinent. MDFT therapists link parents' alcohol and substance use to their parenting deficits, highlighting how alcohol use impairs their ability to be consistent, firm, and available to their child. Therapists help parents access mental health and substance abuse services to address their own needs. Individual sessions with the parent(s) include discussion of parenting philosophy and practices, assessing skills in implementing core parenting skills such as monitoring, limit setting, and communicating to the adolescent age appropriate maturity demands.

With this foundation in place, productive work can be done in family sessions to heal past hurts related to the parents' drinking and commit to helping each other achieve and maintain sobriety. As a result of individual work with the adolescent to explore his or her disappointment, shame, and anger related to the parents' drinking, many youth are prepared to share some of these experiences and feelings in family sessions. These family sessions can be very powerful motivators for parents to take steps toward their own recovery. These discussions are often empowering for teens as well, in that years of pent-up emotions can be shared and families can move toward forgiveness and a commitment to help each other in the recovery process.

Family-Based Relapse Prevention

The study of relapse trajectories following alcohol treatment has shed light on the different patterns of alcohol use and predictors and consequences of relapse after treatment (Chung and Maisto, 2006). Research shows that following standard outpatient treatment in the community, the medium time to relapse with alcohol is only 26 days, using the most stringent criteria for defining relapse, and between one-half and two-thirds of youth relapse by the 6 month follow-up (Cornelius et al., 2003). Alcohol use plays an important role in relapse among teens following treatment, even among those who do not report alcohol use as their substance of choice at intake (Brown et al., 2002). Protective factors against relapse include aftercare participation, better alcohol coping skills, and positive supports for recovery (Chung et al., 2004). Understanding different relapse trajectories has helped identify those youth who may need more intensive treatment and follow-up services. Taken together, these studies underscore the importance of bolstering coping and relapse prevention skills during treatment and providing continued support for abstinence and following the formal treatment phase.

Family functioning has been found to play a primary role in helping teens achieve and maintain abstinence. For instance, parental participation in youth substance abuse treatment predicts positive outcomes at both 6 and 12 months (Hsieh et al., 1998). Improvements in family relationships are strongly related to long-term maintenance of treatment goals following adolescent substance abuse treatment (Brown et al., 1994), whereas family drug use is linked to poorer treatment retention and more alcohol use among teens after treatment (Galaif et al., 2001). Further, firm family rules and consequences about drinking both related to initial motivation to stop drinking and predicted taking action to change drinking behaviors 3 months following adolescents' alcohol-related medical emergencies (Barnett et al., 2002). Families are clearly important in maintaining post-treatment gains.

In MDFT, individual sessions with teens focus on the context, meaning, and consequences of drinking so that positive alternatives can be generated and adopted. In contrast to more traditional family therapy models, MDFT directly and systematically targets the drinking and related cognitions and behaviors, rather than assuming drinking will abate when family conflict reduces and parents become more effective in implementing positive parenting strategies. The MDFT therapist helps teens recognize the emotional, behavioral, and cognitive antecedents to drinking, and to identify the consequences of drinking in relation to problems with family members, peers, school, and the legal system (as well as longer-term ramifications if the use continues). Drinking is considered a problem not from a moralistic or legalistic standpoint, but because excessive drinking keeps adolescents from reaching the goals they have set for themselves. Regular drinking keeps teens from being available to themselves to make good decisions about their lives. Progress in avoiding friends and situations where they will be tempted to drink and using coping skills generated in individual sessions is continually linked back to the teens' stated hopes and dreams for themselves. In this way, motivation is elicited for long-term abstinence beyond the completion of therapy.

In addition to individual work, family interventions are aimed at promoting new interactional patterns among family members. Since the family environment is an important context of adolescent functioning, and communication and interactions are generally compromised in substance abusing families, the family interactional realm is generally in need of significant attention during treatment and following the initial treatment phase. One of the goals of MDFT is to create a new family environment in which the family becomes the therapeutic agent long after the MDFT therapist has completed work with the teen and parents. Thus MDFT family sessions use the technique of enactment to elicit and shape discussions of important topics, including substance use and ways to cope with drinking urges. These interventions provide *in vivo* opportunities for the therapist to take an active and directive stance toward the prompting of new responses and supportive behaviors from family members. Issues raised in the individual sessions with the parents and with the teenager are brought into the family meetings, with the encouragement, support, and facilitation of the therapist.

A complementary component of work that helps to maintain the teen's recovery during and following treatment is in the extrafamilial realm. MDFT therapists aim to improve the parents' and adolescent's functioning relative to important and influential social systems outside of the family and to promote the adolescent's involvement in prosocial activities. For instance, therapists contact school and arrange meetings, coaching the parents and adolescents about what is required in these situations to facilitate the best possible outcomes, and how to maintain good outcomes after treatment. The fundamental premise of extrafamilial interventions is that changes in parents, adolescents, and in family interactions are insufficient unless social environment factors and realities are taken into account. Extrafamilial interventions facilitate a new kind of mindset and competence of parents and adolescents vis a vis these developmentally influential social systems, promoting additional supports for abstinence following the end of treatment. For example, added support during and following treatment is facilitated by encouraging adolescents' participation in teen-focused AA meetings. Multiple-systems oriented approaches such as MDFT have the advantage of addressing intrapersonal, social, familial, and extrafamilial relapse risk factors.

EMPIRICAL SUPPORT FOR MDFT WITH ADOLESCENT ALCOHOL ABUSERS

Examining results of Multidimensional Family Therapy with adolescent drug abusers who also reported alcohol use suggests that the model has promise with teen drinkers. For instance, in the first trial of MDFT, the model was compared to two other standard, once-a-week (14-16 sessions), office-based therapies (adolescent group therapy and multifamily education) with a sample of youth who were almost all combinational users of both alcohol and marijuana (Liddle et al., 2001). At termination, youth assigned to MDFT showed a 54% reduction in combinational alcohol and marijuana use in comparison with only an 18% reduction for group therapy and a 24% reduction for multifamily therapy. The general pattern of results shows the greatest improvement among youth in MDFT, with gains maintained at 6 and 12-mth follow-ups.

Another controlled trial compared MDFT to individual Cognitive Behavior Therapy (CBT) with a primarily male, African American sample with marijuana use disorders (Liddle, 2002b). Examining only those teens who reported drinking at intake (40%) revealed a significant decrease from intake to 12 months following discharge for both the individual (CBT) and family-based (MDFT) treatment conditions. Overall, both treatments reduced symptoms from intake to termination across all three target domains of functioning: substance use, externalizing symptoms, and internalizing symptoms; however, only MDFT was able to maintain treatment gains in these areas after termination and up to the 12-month follow-up.

A third randomized trial compared MDFT with a manualized peer group therapy for drug abusing young adolescents (ages 11-15) who were predominantly male and minority (Liddle et al., 2004). Significant treatment effects (pre-post treatment) were found to favor MDFT in four major risk domains: externalizing symptoms, family cohesion, peer delinquency, and school behavior. In addition, MDFT was more effective than group treatment in decreasing alcohol use in the subset of adolescents who reported drinking at intake (20% of the sample). MDFT participants showed a 71% decrease in alcohol use compared to a 39% *increase* in alcohol use among youth in group treatment from intake to discharge. Youth in MDFT were also more likely to be abstinent from alcohol at the 12 month follow-up than teens in group treatment.

In a series of clinical trials, MDFT has demonstrated more significant reductions in the target symptoms of substance abuse, internalizing and externalizing symptoms, delinquency, school performance, and family problems than comparison treatments. There is also evidence that MDFT can reduce alcohol use and maintain these gains up to 12 months after therapy.

CONCLUSIONS

We have presented an empirically based justification and outline for new areas of treatment development for MDFT with adolescent alcohol abusers. The treatment development work that has been done in the family-based specialty generally and in MDFT specifically has focused mainly on drug abusing samples. This specialty area is poised for breakthroughs with alcohol abusing teens if careful theoretically and empirically based treatment development work is done. The theory that guides this work is based on a thorough understanding of the known determinants, ingredients, and contextual factors that predict alcohol problems among teens.

With sound theory, preliminary outcomes, and a vast empirical base on risk factors to guide the implementation of family-based alcohol-specific interventions for teens, rigorous study of these approaches with drinking samples is an important next step. Many questions remain unresolved regarding differences among teens with comorbid drug and alcohol use disorders versus those with primary abuse of alcohol. As noted above, the etiological pathways to different substance use disorders may be different, suggesting that interventions may need to be alcohol-specific. This article outlines promising targets of change with teen drinkers and their families.

REFERENCES

Azrin, N. H., Donohue, B. C., Besalel, V. A., Kogan, E., & Acierno, R. (1994). A new role for psychology in the treatment of drug abuse. *Psychotherapy Private Practice* 13:73-80.

Barnett, N. P., Lebeau-Craven, R. C., O'Leary, T. A., Colby, S. M., Wollard, R., Rohsenow, D.J. et al. (2002). Predictors of motivation to change after medical treatment for drinking-related events in adolescents. *Psychology of Addictive Behaviors* 16:106-1120.

Blanton, H., Gibbons, F. X., Gerrard, M., Conger, K. J. and Smith, G. E. (1997). Role of family and peers in the development of prototypes associated with substance use. *Journal of Family Psychology* 11:271-288.

Brody, G. H., Ge, X., Katz, J. and Arias, I. (2000). A longitudinal analysis of internalization of parental alcohol-use norms and adolescent alcohol use. *Journal of Applied Developmental Science* 4:71-79.

Brown, T. G., Seraganian, P., Tremblay, J. and Annis, H. (2002). Matching substance abuse aftercare treatments to client characteristics. *Addictive Behaviors* 27(4):585-604.

Brown, S. A., Myers, M. G., Mott, M. A. & Vik, P.W. (1994). Correlates of success following treatment for adolescent substance abuse. *Applied and Preventive Psychology* 3:6173.

Chassin, R. A., Fora, D. B., & King, K. M. (2004). Trajectories of alcohol and drug use and dependency from adolescence to adulthood: The effects of familial alcoholism and personality. *Journal of Abnormal Psychology* 113(4):483-498.

Chassin, L., Curran, P. C., Hussong, A. M., & Colder, C. R. (1996). The relation of parent alcoholism to adolescent substance use: A longitudinal follow-up study. *Journal of Abnormal Psychology* 105:70-80.

Chung, T. & Maisto, S. A. (2006). Relapse to alcohol and other drug use in treated adolescents: Review and reconsideration of relapse as a change point in clinical course. *Clinical Psychology Review* 26(2):149-61.

Chung, T., Maisto, S. A., Cornelius, J. R., & Martin, C. S. (2004). Adolescents' alcohol and drug use trajectories in the year following treatment. *Journal of Studies on Alcohol* 65(1):105-114.

Colder, C. R. & Chassin, L. (1999). The psychosocial characteristics of alcohol users versus problem users: Data from a study of adolescents at risk. *Developmental Psychopathology* 11(2):321–348.

Communities That Care. (2004). "Prevention Strategies Guide" http://www.channingbete.com/positiveyouth/pages/CTC/CTC.html

Cornelius, J. R., Maisto, S. A., Pollock, N. K., Martin, C. S., Salloum, I. M., Lynch, K. G. et al. (2003). Rapid relapse generally follows treatment for substance use disorders among adolescents. *Addictive Behaviors* 28(2):381-386.

Center for Substance Abuse Treatment (CSAT). (1998). *Treatment of adolescents with substance use disorders.* Treatment Improvement Protocol (TIP) Series, Number 32. DHHS Pub. no. (SMA) 01-3494. Washington, DC: U.S. Government Printing Office.

Diamond, G. M., Liddle, H. A., Hogue, A. & Dakof, G. A. (2000). Alliance building interventions with adolescents in family therapy: A process study. *Psychotherapy: Theory, Research, Practice & Training* 36(4):355-368.

Dishion, T. J. & Medici-Skaggs, N. (2000). An ecological analysis of monthly "bursts" in early adolescent substance use. *Journal of Applied Developmental Science* 4(2):89-97.

Drug Strategies. (2003). "Treating Teens: A Guide to Adolescent Drug Programs" http://www.drugstrategies.org/teen; and http://www.npr.org/programs/atc/features/2003/mar/treating_teens/miami_treatment_program.pdf

Ellis, D. A., Rucker, A. & Fitzgerald, H. E. (1997). The role of family influences in development and risk. *Alcohol Health and Research World* 21:218-226.

Fitzgerald, H. E., Sullivan, L. A., Ham, H. P. and Zucker, R. A. (1993). Predictors of behavior problems in the three-year-old sons of alcoholics: Early evidence for the onset of risk. *Child Development* 64:110-123.

Garnier, H. E. and Stein, J. A. (2002). An 18-year model of family and peer effects on adolescent drug use and delinquency. *Journal of Youth and Adolescence* 31:45-56.

Grant, J. D., Scherrer, J. F., Lynskey, M. T., Lyons, M. J, Eisen, S. A, Tsuan, M. T., True, W. R. Guilamo, R., Jaccard, V., Turrisi, J., Johansson, R. and Alida, M.B. (2006). Maternal perceptions of alcohol use by adolescents who drink alcohol. *Journal of Studies on Alcohol* 67(5):730-737.

Guo, J., Hawkins, J. D., Hill, K.G. and Abbott, R. D. (2001). Childhood and adolescent predictors of alcohol abuse and dependence in young adulthood. *Journal of Studies on Alcohol* 62:754-762.

Havey, J. M. and Dodd, D. K. (1995). Children of alcoholics, negative life events and early experimentation with drugs. *Journal of School Psychology* 33(4):305-317.

Henggeler, S. W. (1999). Multisystemic therapy: An overview of clinical procedures, outcomes, and policy implications. *Child Psychology and Psychiatry Review* 4(1):2-10.

Henggeler, S. W., Pickrel, S. G. and Brondino, M. J. (1999). Multisystemic treatment of substance abusing and dependent delinquents: Outcomes, treatment fidelity and transportability. *Mental Health Service Research* 1:171-184.

Henggeler, S. W., Borduin, C. M., Melton, G. B., Mann, B. J., Smith, L. A. and Hall, J. A. (1991). Effects of multisystemic therapy on drug use and abuse in serious juvenile offenders: A progress report from two outcome studies. *Family Dynamics of Addiction Quarterly* 1:40-51.

Hogue, A., Liddle, H.A., Becker, D. and Johnson-Leckrone, J. (2002). Family-based prevention counseling for high-risk young adolescents: Immediate outcomes. *Journal of Community Psychology* 30:1-22.

Hsieh, S., Hoffmann, N. G., and Hollister, C. D. (1998). The relationship between pre-, during-, post-treatment factors and adolescent substance abuse behaviors. *Addictive Behaviors* 23:477-488.

Hussong, A. M., Curran, P. J. Chassin, L. (1998). Pathways of risk for accelerated heavy alcohol use among adolescent children of alcoholic parents. *Journal of Abnormal Psychology* 26:453-466.

Hussong, A. M. and Chassin, L. (1997). Substance use initiation among adolescent children of alcoholics: Testing protective factors. *Journal of Studies on Alcohol* 58:272-279.

Institute of Medicine. (1990). Broadening the base for treatment of alcohol problems. Washington, DC: National Academy Press.

Jackson-Gilfort, A., Liddle, H. A., Tejeda, M. J. and Dakof, G. A. (2001). Facilitating engagement of African American male adolescents in family therapy: A cultural theme process study. *Journal of Black Psychology* 27:321-340.

Kazdin, A. E. (1994). Methodology, design and evaluation in psychotherapy research. In *Handbook of psychotherapy and behavior change,* eds. Bergin AE and Garfield SL, 19-71. New York: John Wiley & Sons.

Kelley, M. L. and Fals-Stewart, W. (2002). Couples-versus individual based therapy for alcohol and drug abuse: Effects on children's psychosocial functioning. *The Journal of Consulting and Clinical Psychology* 70:417-427.

Kuntsche, E. N. and Kuendig, H. (2006). What is worse? A hierarchy of family-related risk factors predicting alcohol use in adolescence. *Substance Use and Misuse* 41(1): 71-86.

Kuperman, S., Schlosser, S. S., Lidral, J. and Reich, W. (1999). Relationship of child psychopathology to parental alcoholism and antisocial personality disorder. *Journal of the American Academy of Child & Adolescent Psychiatry* 38:686-692.

Liddle, H. A. (2004). Family-based therapies for adolescent alcohol and drug abuse: research contributions and future research needs. *Addiction* 99(2):76-92.

Liddle, H. A., Rowe, C. L., Henderson, C., Dakof, G. A. and Ungaro, R. A. (2004). Early intervention for adolescent substance abuse: Pretreatment to posttreatment outcomes of a randomized controlled trial comparing multidimensional family therapy and peer group treatment. *Journal of Psychoactive Drugs* 36(1):2-37.

Liddle, H. A. (2002a). *Multidimensional Family Therapy Treatment (MDFT) for Adolescent Cannabis Users*. Rockville, MD: Center for Substance Abuse Treatment, Substance Abuse and Mental Health Services Administration.

Liddle, H. A. (2002b). Advances in family-based therapy for adolescent substance abuse: Findings from the Multidimensional Family Therapy research program. In *Problems of drug dependence 2001: Proceedings of the 63rd annual scientific meeting* ed. Harris LS, 113-115. Bethesda, MD: National Institute on Drug Abuse.

Liddle, H. A., Dakof G. A., Parker, K., Diamond, G. S., Barrett. K. and Tejeda, M. (2001). Multidimensional family therapy for adolescent substance abuse: Results of a randomized clinical trial. *American Journal of Drug Alcohol Abuse* 27:651-687.

Lowman, C. (2004). Developing effective evidence-based interventions for adolescents with alcohol use disorders. *Journal of Addiction* 99(s2):1-4.

Maisto, S. A., Pollock, N. K., Cornelius, J. R., Lynch, K. G. and Martin, C. S. (2003). Alcohol relapse as a function of relapse definition in a clinical sample of adolescents. *Addictive Behaviors* 28(3):449-459.

Maisto, S. A., Pollock, N. K., Kaczynski, N. A., Lynch, K. G. and Martin, C. S. (2001). Course of functioning in adolescents 1 year after alcohol and other drug treatment. *Psychology of Addictive Behavior* 15:68-76.

McGue, M. (1997). A behavioral-genetic perspective on children of alcoholics. *Alcohol Health and Research World* 21(3):210-217.

National Institute on Drug Abuse (NIDA). (1999). *Scientifically based approaches to drug addiction treatment. In Principles of Drug Addiction Treatment: A research-based guide*. (Rep. No. NIH publication No. 99-4180, pp. 35-47). Rockville, MD: NIDA.

O'Farrell, T. J. and Fals-Stewart, W. (2003). Alcohol abuse. *Journal of Marital Family Therapy* 29(1):121-146.

Perry, C. L., Williams, C. L., Veblen-Mortenson, S., Toomey, T. L., Komro, K. A., Anstine, P. S. et al. (1996). Project Northland: Outcomes of a community-wide alcohol use prevention program during early adolescence. *American Journal of Public Health* 86:956-965.

Rigter, H., Van Gageldonk, A. and Ketelaars, T. (2004). *Treatment and other interventions targeting drug use and addiction: State of the art 2004.* Utrecht: National Drug Monitor.

Rowe, C. L., and Liddle, H. A. (2003). Substance abuse. *Journal of Marital Family Therapy* 29:97-120.

Rowe, C. L., Parker-Sloat, B., Schwartz, S. and Liddle, H. L. (2003). Family therapy for early adolescent substance abuse. In *Adolescent substance abuse treatment in the United States: Exemplary models from a national evaluation study, eds.* Stevens SJ and Morral AR, 105-132.

Sher, K. J., Gotham, H. J. and Watson, A. L. (2004). Trajectories of dynamic predictors of disorders: Their meanings and implications. *Development and Psychopathology Fall* 16(4):825-856.

Sher, K. J. (1994). Individual-level risk factors. In *The development of alcohol problems: Exploring the biopsychosocial matrix of risk,* eds. Zucker, R., Boyd, G. and Howard, J., 77-108. U.S. Department of Health and Human Services, Public Health Service National Institute of Health

Sher, K. J., Walitzer, K. S., Wood, P. K. and Brent, E. E. (1991). Characteristics of children of alcoholics' putative risk factors, substance use and abuse, and psychopathology. *Journal of Abnormal Psychology* 100:427-448.

Stanton, M. D. and Shadish, W. R. (1997). Outcome, attrition, and family–couples treatment for drug abuse: A meta-analysis and review of the controlled, comparative studies. *Psychological Bulletin* 122:170-191.

Stice, E., Myers, M. G. and Brown, S. A. (1998). A longitudinal grouping analysis of adolescent substance use escalation and de-escalation. *Psychology of Addictive Behaviors* 12:14-27.

Tapert, S. F., Cheung, E. H., Brown, G. G., Frank, L. R., Paulus, M. P., Schweinsburg, A. D. et al. (2003). Neural responses to alcohol stimuli in adolescents with alcohol use disorder. *Archives of General Psychiatry* 60(7):727-735.

Trepper, T. S., Piercy, F.P., Lewis, R. A., Volk, R. J. and Sprenkle, D.H. (1993). Family therapy for adolescent alcohol abuse. In *Treating alcohol problems: marital and family interventions.* ed. O'Farrell TJ, 261-278. New York, NY: Guilford Press.

Van Zundert Rinka, M. P., Van Der Vorst, H., Vermulst Ad, A. and Engels, R. CME. (2006). Pathways to alcohol use among Dutch students in regular education and education for adolescents with behavioral problems: The role of parental alcohol use, general parenting practices, and alcohol-specific parenting practices. *Journal of Family Psychology* 20(3):456-467.

Weinberg, N. Z., Dielman, T. E., Mandell, W. and Shope, J. T. (1994). Parental drinking and gender factors in the prediction of early adolescent alcohol use. *International Journal of the Addictions* 29:89–104.

Windle, M. (1996). Effect of parental drinking on adolescents. *Alcohol Research and Health* 20:181-184.

Zhou, Q., King, K. M. and Chassin, L. (2006). The roles of familial alcoholism and adolescent family harmony in young adults' substance dependence disorders: Mediated and moderated relations. *Journal of Abnormal Psychology* 115(2):320-331.

Zucker, R. A. (1994). Pathways to alcohol problems and alcoholism: a developmental account of the evidence for multiple alcoholisms and for contextual contributions to risk. In *The development of alcohol problems: Exploring the biopsychosocial matrix of risk,* eds. Zucker, R., Boyd, G. and Howard, J., 255-289. Rockville, MD: NIH.

doi:10.1300/J020v26n01_06

Multisystemic Therapy
for Alcohol and Other Drug Abuse
in Delinquent Adolescents

Ashli J. Sheidow, PhD
Scott W. Henggeler, PhD

SUMMARY. Multisystemic Therapy (MST) has been identified as an effective treatment of youth antisocial behavior, including substance abuse. This article provides an overview of the clinical application of MST, focusing on its implementation with alcohol and other drug using adolescents, and summarizes findings from clinical trials using MST to treat substance use disorders in adolescents. doi:10.1300/J020v26n01_07

Ashli J. Sheidow is Assistant Professor, Family Services Research Center, Department of Psychiatry and Behavioral Sciences, Medical University of South Carolina.

Scott W. Henggeler is Director, Family Services Research Center and Professor, Department of Psychiatry and Behavioral Sciences.

Address correspondence to: Ashli J. Sheidow, PhD, Department of Psychiatry and Behavioral Sciences, Medical University of South Carolina, 67 President Street, Charleston, SC 29425 (E-mail: sheidoaj@musc.edu).

Website address for the MST program at the Family Services Research Center is: http://www.musc.edu/psychiatry/research/fsrc/mst.htm.

This manuscript was supported by grants K23DA015658, R01DA08029, R01DA 10079, R01DA08029, and R01DA13066 from the National Institute on Drug Abuse and by grant R01AA122202 from the National Institute on Alcoholism and Alcohol Abuse and the Center for Substance Abuse Treatment.

[Haworth co-indexing entry note]: "Multisystemic Therapy for Alcohol and Other Drug Abuse in Delinquent Adolescents." Sheidow, Ashli J., and Scott W. Henggeler. Co-published simultaneously in *Alcoholism Treatment Quarterly* (The Haworth Press) Vol. 26, No. 1/2, 2008, pp. 125-145; and: *Family Intervention in Substance Abuse: Current Best Practices* (ed: Oliver J. Morgan, and Cheryl H. Litzke) The Haworth Press, 2008, pp. 125-145. Single or multiple copies of this article are available for a fee from The Haworth Document Delivery Service [1-800-HAWORTH, 9:00 a.m. - 5:00 p.m. (EST). E-mail address: docdelivery@haworthpress. com].

KEYWORDS. Treatment, multisystemic therapy, adolescent, alcohol-other drug abuse, juvenile delinquency

INTRODUCTION

The evidence base for Multisystemic Therapy (MST; Henggeler, Schoenwald, Borduin, Rowland, & Cunningham, 1998) spans the past two decades and includes publication of nine randomized clinical trials and one quasi-experimental study with adolescents presenting serious antisocial behavior and their families. Based on findings from this body of clinical research, MST has been identified as an effective treatment of youth antisocial behavior, including substance abuse (National Institute on Drug Abuse, 1999; President's New Freedom Commission on Mental Health, 2003; U.S. Public Health Service, 2001). This article provides an overview of the clinical application of MST, focusing on its implementation with substance using adolescents, and summarizes findings from clinical trials using MST to treat substance use disorders in adolescents.

THEORETICAL AND EMPIRICAL BASES OF MST

The MST model, which focuses on youths with serious antisocial behavior who are at imminent risk of costly out-of-home placements and their families, was shaped by general systems theory (von Bertalanffy, 1968) and Bronfenbrenner's (1979) theory of social ecology. Major tenets of these theories are that behavior is multidetermined and bidirectional in nature. Importantly, these theoretical frameworks have been supported by developmental research on the correlates and causes of adolescent behavior problems, where risk and protective factors have been identified across individual, family, peer, school, and community contexts (e.g., Hawkins et al., 1998; Weinberg, Rahdert, Colliver, & Glantz, 1998). Thus, guided by ecological and systems theory as well as extant risk factor research, the MST assessment process and intervention protocols focus on individual, family, peer, school, and social network variables that are linked with identified problems as well as on the interface of these systems.

CLINICAL PROCEDURES

MST intervention protocols are relatively complex in light of the multiple determinants of antisocial behavior, the serious and interrelated problems presented by youthful offenders and their families, and the array of evidence-based interventions that can be used. Consequently, considerable resources have been devoted to specifying MST treatment protocols and to developing strategies to support practitioner implementation fidelity. A brief overview of clinical procedures with some examples and a sample case are provided here, but the reader is referred to the extensive body of MST empirical and descriptive literature. In particular, Henggeler and colleagues have described MST clinical procedures in detail for treating adolescent antisocial behavior (Henggeler et al., 1998) and serious emotional disturbance (Henggeler, Schoenwald, Rowland, & Cunningham, 2002). Many case examples are provided in these clinical volumes, and chapters are devoted to the development and implementation of interventions for difficulties at individual, family, peer, school, and neighborhood (e.g., Swenson, Henggeler, Taylor, & Addison, 2005) levels.

MST Treatment Principles

Given the complexity of cases treated by MST and in contrast with many evidence-based treatment models, MST does not use a "cookbook" or "checklist" approach; that is, treatment is individualized such that each case receives a set of interventions tailored to the strengths and weaknesses of the youth and his or her family. The design of MST clinical procedures is operationalized through nine core principles that guide assessment practices, treatment planning, and the integration of evidence-based interventions. MST therapists and supervisors apply these principles within a standardized analytical/decision making process (described subsequently) that structures and individualizes treatment planning, implementation, and evaluation. Throughout all aspects of planning and conducting treatment, the supervisor and team follow the nine principles of MST. These principles are listed in italics in Table 1, and a corresponding description and example(s) follow each.

TABLE 1. Multisystemic Therapy Treatment Principles

1.   FINDING THE FIT

The primary purpose of assessment is to understand the "fit" between the identified problems and their broader systemic context. Utilizing what we know about the correlates and causes of youth problems, MST providers conceptualize youth and family symptoms from an ecological, systemic perspective. Thus, using the MST Analytic Process, clinicians investigate and target for treatment "fit factors," or characteristics of the youth's ecology that are maintaining the problem behavior (see sample case for examples). Notably, the assessment process is dynamic throughout treatment, with regular monitoring of progress and updating of newly identified or appropriately resolved fit factors.

2.   POSITIVE AND STRENGTH FOCUSED

Therapeutic contacts emphasize the positive and use systemic strengths as levers for change. Clinicians maintain a strength focused and optimistic perspective that is communicated clearly to the family throughout the assessment and treatment process. This optimism is supported overtly through supervision and peer consultation. Providers identify strengths within the various ecological contexts, investigating child factors (e.g., competencies, attractiveness, altruism), caregiver factors (e.g., resources, affective bonds, social support), peer factors (e.g., competencies, prosocial activities), school factors (e.g., management practices, concern, prosocial activities), and neighborhood or community factors (e.g., law enforcement, business involvement, healthcare, neighbor concern). Identified strengths are then utilized in interventions. For instance, if low monitoring during afterschool hours is contributing to the adolescent's involvement in antisocial behavior, then monitoring may be partially addressed by empowering the caregiver to engage the youth in organized, prosocial activities available at the school or in the community. Importantly, clinicians are trained to incorporate this strength-based approach throughout their work. For instance, supervisors assist clinicians in identifying "barriers" to treatment success rather than perceiving clients as being resistant to change.

3.   INCREASING RESPONSIBILITY

Interventions are designed to promote responsible behavior and decrease irresponsible behavior among family members. Providers view parents as a primary lever for change. Rather than providing individual treatment for the youth, providers empower caregivers to bring about changes in the youth's behavior and within the youth's ecology. For example, caregivers may be instructed in basic behavioral techniques such as spelling out rules and contingencies, and appropriately enforcing the contingency plan. Further, youth are directed to take responsibility for their behavior through this process by having input into the contingency plan.

4. PRESENT-FOCUSED, ACTION-ORIENTED, AND WELL-DEFINED

Interventions are present-focused and action-oriented, targeting specific and well-defined problems. This principle is tied closely with assessment in that treatment goals are determined through a collaborative effort among the provider, caregivers, youth, and other key players in the youth's ecology (e.g., teacher, probation officer). These clearly stated goals are then translated into an explicit treatment plan in which the MST treatment team integrates pragmatic, ecologically minded interventions. This plan is monitored closely to ensure that treatment is making quantifiable progress in improving identified problems. As a result, treatment is highly focused and geared toward swift improvement in and resolution of symptoms.

5. TARGETING SEQUENCES

Interventions target sequences of behavior within or between multiple systems that maintain the identified problems. This principle also is tied closely to assessment in that identified problems are conceptualized from a social ecological perspective, and this conceptualization guides treatment decisions. For example, an identified problem behavior within the school may be maintained, in part, because the behavior is not being consequented in a timely and systematic manner at home. If the clinician discovers this lack of consequenting is due to a pattern of hostile or derogatory interactions the clinician between the caregiver and the school that has reduced the effectiveness of communication, the clinician might aim to alter communication between the caregiver and the school as a means of improving behavioral contingencies and resultant youth behavior.

6. DEVELOPMENTALLY APPROPRIATE

Interventions are developmentally appropriate and fit the developmental needs of the youth. MST individualizes treatment to the developmental stage of a youth and family. For instance, cognitive interventions might be more suited to an older adolescent who has the ability to monitor and process cognitions than to a preteen who might have less capacity for such tasks. Another example of tailoring treatment to the developmental needs of the youth is in peer interventions. An adolescent has increased need for independence and autonomy from the family and should be allowed and encouraged to maintain peer relationships. However, this peer interaction should be monitored and directed by caregivers to prevent interaction with negative peers and promote interaction with prosocial peers.

7. CONTINUOUS EFFORT

Interventions are designed to require daily or weekly effort by family members. After adequately engaging families, MST clinicians provide treatment in a manner that is meant to bring about rapid change. Because clinicians collaborate with the caregivers, the youth, and other key players in the youth's ecology to identify and define treatment

TABLE 1 (continued)

goals, these participants are expected, and supported, to share the responsibility in achieving these goals. This participation must be intensive (i.e., daily or weekly) to bring about rapid and acute change in youth problems, with families learning that they are the "change agents" (i.e., they become empowered to bring about change).

8. EVALUATION AND ACCOUNTABILITY

Intervention effectiveness is evaluated continuously from multiple perspectives with providers assuming accountability for overcoming barriers to successful outcomes. As mentioned earlier, assessment within MST is a dynamic process that circularly informs treatment. Because goals are well-defined, measurable outcomes can be monitored. Frequent checks of treatment progress assist clinicians in identifying and targeting barriers to treatment success. MST clinicians are trained to hold themselves accountable for treatment progress rather than deeming a family or youth at fault for a lack of success. Clinicians are taught to "never give up" on a youth or family, but instead to identify the barriers to success and to develop means to overcome those barriers.

9. GENERALIZATION

Interventions are designed to promote treatment generalization and long-term maintenance of therapeutic change by empowering caregivers to address family members' needs across multiple systemic contexts. Caregivers are viewed as the key to maintaining treatment successes, and much effort is spent helping caregivers to develop the skills necessary for continuing the progress made during treatment. For example, a care giver might be instructed on the use of simple cognitive-behavioral or problem-solving techniques so that he or she may help guide the youth through such exercises without the presence of the clinician. Importantly, caregivers are also surrounded by indigenous supports(e.g., extended family, neighbors, friends) to help sustain favorable outcomes. Thus, the interventions that occur within MST are integrated in a way that will support long-term maintenance of treatment progress.

Many of these principles represent a remarkable departure from the usual services families encounter today. As conveyed in principles 1, 4 and 8, MST relies heavily on thorough and careful assessment procedures both initially and throughout treatment, with the clinicians taking responsibility for assuring case progress (by overcoming the barriers of the family and ecology). In addition, these continuous assessment procedures ensure highly focused and individualized interventions so therapeutic progress can be achieved as quickly as possible (consistent with principles 4 and 7). Guided by principle 2, MST clinicians make every effort to avoid blaming language and, consistent with principles 3 and 9, generate creative ways to empower caregivers and other naturally occurring supports in the ecology. These principles are effectively integrated throughout treatment via the MST Analytical Process, described next, and the extensive support system employed in delivering MST.

MST Analytic Process

The MST analytical process (see Figure 1) outlines the procedures by which youth and family problems are prioritized and targeted for change. After receiving the referral, along with a description of the referral behaviors, the therapist's first objective is to rapidly obtain engagement and alignment with the youth's family and other key participants in the family's social ecology (e.g., extended family, neighbors and friends, school and teachers, juvenile justice authorities and probation officers). Following MST Principle 8, the therapist and team take responsibility for creating and sustaining this environment of Alignment and Engagement and must sometimes be creative in doing so (e.g., meeting with a teacher over lunch, conversing with a coach while helping to set up practice equipment). While establishing such engagement, the therapist obtains the desired outcomes from each of the key participants, ensuring that the outcome is defined in specific, measurable terms (e.g., attending school, abstaining from cannabis use). The MST therapist and family next convert the key participants' desired outcomes and referral behaviors into a set of overarching goals of treatment (usually three to four Overarching Goals), with each goal having a measurable outcome defined by the key participants.

The next step in the Analytical Process moves the therapist and MST team into the hypothesis testing procedure utilized in MST, informally called the "Do-Loop." Based on multiple perspectives (e.g., opinions of stakeholders, clinical impressions, research derived knowledge), the ecological factors that seem to be driving or sustaining each problem behavior (e.g., low monitoring of youth's activities and whereabouts, ineffective contingencies employed by caregivers, involvement with negative peers who provide access to drugs and places to use) are organized into a coherent conceptual framework. This is referred to as finding the "fit" of the problem, and fit factors are prioritized in a systematic manner to identify the initial targets of intervention (i.e., those determinants of antisocial behavior that are more powerful and proximal). This analysis results in a working hypothesis about how best to change the youth's problem behavior, and the working hypothesis is used to generate the Intermediary Goals of treatment (e.g., the therapist and family will develop clear rules, rewards, and consequences that the caregiver can implement consistently). Next, the MST therapist, with

FIGURE 1. Multisystemic Therapy (MST) Analytical Process

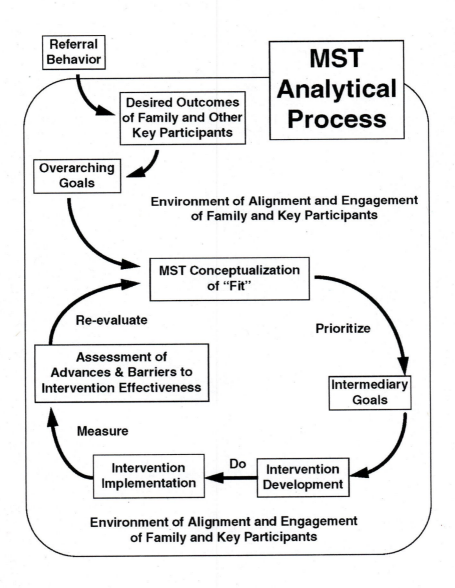

support from other team members, the MST supervisor, and an MST expert consultant, designs specific intervention strategies to target the prioritized fit factors by adapting empirically-based interventions from pragmatic, problem-focused treatments that have at least some empirical support. In deciding on which specific interventions to use, the individual strengths and needs of the youth, family, and their social network are considered to maximize the odds of success (see MST Principle 2). Selected interventions might include techniques from strategic family therapy (Haley, 1987), structural family therapy (Minuchin, 1974), behavioral parent training (Munger, 1993), and cognitive behavior therapies (Kendall & Braswell, 1993).

As denoted on the left-hand side of the "Do-Loop" and MST Principle 8, outcomes of the intervention(s) are evaluated each week to determine advances and barriers (e.g., low engagement, poor implementation of intervention) to intervention effectiveness. Favorable and unfavorable results are used to improve conceptualization of the fit for the youth's problem behaviors and a corresponding revision of hypotheses. Through this recursive feedback process, ineffective interventions are reconceptualized and modifications are made until effective strategies are developed and implemented. Importantly, the MST team holds itself accountable for achieving the goals of treatment and constantly strives for ways to overcome barriers to success.

Treatment Delivery

MST uses a home-based (e.g., home, school, and community settings) model of service delivery to decrease barriers to service access and enhance family engagement. Full-time Master's level therapists work within a team of three to four therapists, and each team is supervised by an advanced Master's level or doctoral level supervisor who devotes at least 50% time to the team. Therapists each carry caseloads of four to six families, and clinicians provide 24-hour/7 day a week availability. This flexible scheduling allows for sessions at convenient times for families and ensures that therapists can respond quickly to crises that might threaten goal attainment (i.e., prevent out-of-home placement). Average length of treatment is 4 to 5 months per family.

Quality Assurance

Several studies have demonstrated significant linkages between therapist adherence to the MST treatment protocols and important clinical outcomes for youths (e.g., Henggeler, Melton, Brondino, Scherer, & Hanley, 1997; Henggeler, Pickrel, & Brondino, 1999; Huey, Henggeler, Brondino, & Pickrel, 2000; Schoenwald, Sheidow, Letourneau, & Liao, 2003). In light of the established importance of treatment fidelity for obtaining desired youth outcomes, the transport of MST programs to provider organizations across the United States and other countries has relied upon a thorough set of quality assurance procedures to support MST practitioners working in community settings. Components of this quality assurance system include: (a) extensive organizational consultation prior to and following the development of MST programs in community-based settings; (b) manualized assessment, intervention, supervision (Henggeler & Schoenwald, 1998), and consultation (Schoenwald, 1998) processes; (c) didactic and experiential training for clinicians, followed by regular booster sessions by MST experts, weekly supervision within the MST treatment team (consisting of therapists and MST supervisor), and weekly consultation with an MST expert; and (d) use of treatment and supervisory fidelity feedback measures including, for example, monthly caregiver reported ratings of therapist adherence on a validated scale. Thus, therapist adherence to the treatment model is monitored continuously, and intensive supports are provided to help therapists achieve optimal outcomes even when facing complex clinical challenges.

Sample Case

Jacob was a 17-year-old youth referred for MST following numerous probation violations, including failure to eliminate alcohol and drug use. He had failed to decrease his substance use following group-based treatment as well as a family-based treatment, and his parents had lost hope that anything would stop him from using drugs. Jacob had started using drugs shortly after his older brother's return home from U.S. military service in the Iraq war. His brother, Jerry, had sustained serious injuries and required pain medication, which Jacob stole to use. Around this same time, Jacob began abusing alcohol with his long-time childhood friends in the hours after school. Jacob's parents both worked fulltime and had been spending most of their free time assisting with Jerry's rehabilitation.

After developing goals for treatment, identifying strengths and weaknesses in the ecology, and conducting a thorough assessment of the factors that appeared to be causing or sustaining Jacob's negative behaviors, the MST therapist began to guide the family in implementing interventions to attenuate Jacob's primary identified problems (i.e., substance abuse, deteriorating school performance, rude and irresponsible behavior at home). For reasons of parsimony, this example focuses on interventions to address Jacob's substance abuse. The first prioritized fit factor (or driver) of the substance abuse was Jacob's easy access to the pain medications. Here, the mother was able to lock Jerry's medications away and track the number of pills consumed. Following this intervention, Jacob ceased his abuse of pain medications, but greatly increased his consumption of alcohol.

. The parents and therapist began to treat the alcohol use by first addressing the driver of "no immediate consequences for use." Because the parents believed they had no way to effectively consequent a 17-year-old, only the probation officer was applying consequences and these were applied infrequently. Using contingency management techniques, Jacob's parents learned how to conduct home tests for drug (urine screens) and alcohol (disposable pipettes) use, and began to test him randomly and when they suspected use (e.g., curfew violation, smell). Based on the test results or if Jacob refused to be tested, Jacob was not allowed to go out for a specified number of nights. In addition, his aggressive reactions to these consequences (e.g., cursing at his parents, punching walls) were assigned increasingly stiffer penalties such as removal of favorite personal possessions (e.g., TV, stereo, computer games, phone). Initially, these contingencies brought about a sharp decline in alcohol use (other substance use did not re-occur, although urine tests continued to ensure he did not begin to use again). However, this success lasted only a few weeks, and Jacob's parents began to withdraw from treatment as they again were frustrated with treatment results and their son's behavior.

To address decreased parental engagement, the therapist increased instrumental support to help the parents manage their older son's rehabilitation as well as the strain on their marital relationship that had developed during the past two years. The therapist also assisted the parents in developing an alternative intervention plan for Jacob. The parents obtained the assistance of Jacob's probation officer to place Jacob on temporary house arrest in lieu of placement. Importantly and in light of the strong negative peer influences experienced by Jacob, the parents informed Jacob that he would have to introduce all his desired friends to his parents and provide phone numbers and addresses so that his parents could meet his friends' parents. Jacob's parents were very reluctant to make these contacts, however, as they were embarrassed to have other community members be aware of their problems. The therapist, consequently, implemented cognitive-behavioral techniques to help the parents evaluate the pros and cons of their options. When the parents decided to follow-through with the peer monitoring plan, the therapist helped them develop and role play strategies for contacting the other parents.

A phased approach to the establishment of appropriate peer relations was used such that Jacob was initially allowed to have approved peers visit him only while his parents were home. The parents arranged to have instrumental supports "pop in" during after school hours to ensure peers were not visiting while Jacob was unsupervised. These indigenous supports included extended family members as well as longtime family friends. After achieving approximately 4 weeks of sobriety, the parents allowed for unsupervised visits by approved peers, with ongoing "pop in" visits for monitoring purposes. The parents realized that Jacob and his friends enjoyed playing poker for entertainment while having these supervised visits–poker recently had become a popular tournament sport broadcast on TV and internet poker games were in vogue. As a reward for continued abstinence, the parents organized a poker party (highly supervised, of course, with rules developed ahead of time and regular checks of all beverages and activities). The party was such a success with Jacob and his friends that the parents continued to have these monthly as Jacob successfully achieved other clinical goals not discussed here (e.g., improved school performance, increased responsibilities at home).

Setbacks, of course, emerged along the way. Jacob came home drunk from a party and his father discovered that Jacob had obtained the beer from the family's own refrigerator. With assistance from the therapist, the parents monitored the alcoholic beverages in the house more closely and began to "pat down" Jacob before he left for parties. On another occasion, Jacob attempted to "play" his parents against one another to avoid accountability, but the improved marital relationship prevented Jacob from being successful. Even with the setbacks, the parents were able to maintain their commitment to the treatment plan due largely to the logic and quality of that plan as well as to their enhanced marital support and assistance from extended family and friends.

EMPIRICAL FINDINGS

MST is regarded as one of the best validated interventions for youths presenting serious clinical problems by federal entities such as the President's New Freedom Commission on Mental Health (2003),

Surgeon General (U.S. Public Health Service, 1999, 2001), National Institute on Drug Abuse (1999), and Center for Substance Abuse Prevention (2001), as well as leading reviewers (e.g., Burns, Hoagwood, & Mrazek, 1999; Elliott, 1998; Farrington & Welsh, 1999; Kazdin & Weisz, 1998; Mihalic, Irwin, Elliott, Fagan, & Hansen, 2001; Stanton & Shadish, 1997). Notably, the Surgeon General (U.S. Public Health Service, 2001) reported MST to be one of only three empirically supported treatments for juvenile offenders, and the Substance Abuse and Mental Health Services Administration (2007) ranks MST as one of their model programs for treatment of this population (see www.modelprograms.samhsa.gov). Findings from MST clinical trials for juvenile offenders are summarized briefly here, concluding with a summary of findings specifically for substance using delinquents.

Empirical Evidence for MST with Delinquent Youth

MST for juvenile delinquency has been the focus of ten published outcome studies. Five randomized trials have been conducted with violent and chronic offenders (Borduin et al., 1995; Henggeler et al., 1997; Henggeler, Melton, & Smith, 1992; Ogden & Halliday-Boykins, 2004; Timmons-Mitchell, Bender, Kishna, & Mitchell, 2006), two with juvenile sexual offenders (Borduin, Henggeler, Blaske, & Stein, 1990; Borduin & Schaeffer, 2001), and two with substance abusing and dependent juvenile offenders (Henggeler, Clingempeel, Brondino, & Pickrel, 2002; Henggeler et al., 2006). A quasi-experimental evaluation was published with inner-city juvenile offenders (Henggeler et al., 1986).

Findings across these studies have consistently favored MST in comparison with control conditions. For example, MST has achieved significant reductions in rates of rearrest and conduct problems across trials, with follow-ups as long as 13.7 years (Schaeffer & Borduin, 2005). Reductions in rates of recidivism have ranged from 26% to 69% across studies for youth treated with MST compared to treated controls. A recent meta-analysis of MST trials (Curtis, Ronan, & Borduin, 2004) included seven outcome studies (708 total participants, 35 MST therapists). Effect sizes averaged .50 for criminal behavior (based on official records), 1.01 for arrest seriousness, and .29 for substance use.

Substance Use Outcomes Within MST Trials

Not surprisingly, extensive evidence supports the strong relationships among adolescent alcohol abuse, drug abuse, and criminal activity (e.g., Crowley, Mikulich, MacDonald, Young, & Zerbe, 1998; Huizinga, Loeber, & Thornberry, 1994). Substance-related outcomes were examined in two of the early randomized trials of MST with violent and chronic juvenile offenders (Borduin et al., 1995; Henggeler et al., 1992). Substance-related findings for MST across both studies were favorable at posttreatment and at 4-year follow-up (Henggeler et al., 1991). Moreover, an almost 14-year follow-up showed that MST participants continued to have fewer drug-related arrests than did treated counterparts (Schaeffer & Borduin, 2005).

Based on the promising findings from the two aforementioned trials with serious juvenile offenders, a study with 118 juvenile offenders meeting DSM-III-R criteria for substance abuse (56%) or dependence (44%) and their families (Henggeler et al., 1999) was conducted. Compared to youth receiving usual community services, youth receiving MST reported lower alcohol and marijuana use at post treatment. Moreover, MST was especially effective at engaging the substance abusing and dependent youths and their families in treatment. Fully 100% (58 of 58) of families in the MST condition were retained for at least 2 months of services, and 98% (57 of 58) were retained until treatment completion at approximately 4 months post referral (Henggeler, Pickrel, Brondino, & Crouch, 1996). These figures are especially remarkable in light of the low client retention rates traditionally attained in the area of substance abuse treatment (Office of Applied Studies, 2000; Stark, 1992).

Findings at 6-month and 4-year follow-ups continued to support the relative effectiveness of MST in this trial, with decreased days incarcerated, decreased total days in out-of-home placement (Schoenwald, Ward, Henggeler, Pickrel, & Patel, 1996), and increased youth attendance in regular school settings (Brown, Henggeler, Schoenwald, Brondino, & Pickrel, 1999) compared to usual services in the 6 months posttreatment. Moreover, cost data showed that the incremental cost of MST was offset by the reduced placement (i.e., incarceration, hospitalization, and residential treatment) of youths in the MST condition (Schoenwald et al., 1996). In the 4-year follow-up (Henggeler, Clingempeel et al., 2002), analyses of drug urine screens demonstrated significantly higher rates of marijuana abstinence for MST participants (55% abstinent) compared to participants who had received usual services (28% abstinent).

A second randomized trial with substance abusing juvenile offenders was completed recently (Henggeler et al., 2006). The purpose of this trial was to determine (a) the effectiveness of juvenile drug court, (b) whether the integration of an evidence-based substance abuse treatment (i.e., MST) into juvenile drug court improved offender outcomes, and

(c) whether the integration of contingency management techniques into MST improved MST substance use outcomes. Contingency management is a well supported substance abuse intervention (Azrin et al., 2001; Petry, 2000) that is theoretically and practically compatible with MST and provides more focused attention on adolescent substance use per se.

In general, findings supported the view that drug court was more effective than family court services in decreasing rates of adolescent-reported substance use and criminal behavior. In addition, findings showed that the use of evidence-based treatments within the drug court context improved youth substance related outcomes. For example, during the first 4 months of drug court participation, 70% of the urine screens were positive for youths in the Drug Court with Community Services condition, in comparison with only 28% and 18% for counterparts in the Drug Court with MST and Drug Court with MST enhanced with Contingency Management conditions, respectively. Urine screens collected over the succeeding 8 months maintained the distinction between Drug Court with Community Services and the Drug Court with MST conditions (45%, 7%, and 17%, respectively). Additional clinical- and cost-related outcomes are being examined in a 5-year follow-up.

In summary, research findings have provided clear support for the effectiveness of MST in treating adolescent substance use problems. MST provides a comprehensive framework that can efficiently integrate specific interventions into a unified, methodical strategy.

CURRENT RESEARCH ON ENHANCING CLINICAL OUTCOMES

MST substance-related research is continuing in several major projects. Bridging clinical and services areas of research, these projects are evaluating adaptations of MST for different clinical populations and studying different strategies for transporting evidence-based substance abuse treatments to community practice settings.

Addressing Parental Substance Abuse

Parental substance abuse is associated with both serious clinical problems in youths (e.g., Hawkins et al., 1998) and families (e.g., National Clearinghouse on Child Abuse and Neglect Information, 2003) and moderates the effectiveness of evidence-based treatments for child behavior problems. Similarly and anecdotally, parents in MST programs who continue to abuse substances often are less equipped to provide effective parenting for their children than are non-substance abusing counterparts. Consequently, two ongoing pilot projects are adapting evidence-based treatments for adult substance abuse for use in MST programs. As described elsewhere in more detail (Schaeffer, Saldana, Rowland, Henggeler, & Swenson, in press), these pilots are adapting the Community Reinforcement Approach (Budney & Higgins, 1998) for use with substance abusing caregivers in families receiving MST and integrating Reinforcement-Based Therapy (Jones, Wong, Tuten, & Stitzer, 2005) with MST adapted to treat child abuse and neglect (Swenson, Saldana et al., 2005).

Comorbid Substance Use and Mental Health Disorders

Rates of psychiatric comorbidity among substance abusing youth are high, and youths with a dual diagnosis are more costly to treat (King, Gaines, Lambert, Summerfelt, & Bickman, 2000). Given the paucity of researched treatments for this population, Sheidow has developed and is evaluating a treatment for dually diagnosed youth that relies on the MST case conceptualization and treatment planning procedures (Sheidow, Molen, Navas-Murphy, & Chapman, 2007). This treatment is directed toward youth in need of an outpatient level of care (traditional MST targets youth who are at imminent risk of out-of-home placement), and provides comprehensive treatment for the co-occurring disorders rather than the sequential or parallel treatments most often used with this population.

Transportability Research

Several studies also are examining the training conditions needed for the effective transport of evidence-based treatments for adolescent substance abuse to community settings. One study is examining the effectiveness of an intensive quality assurance system to promote therapist fidelity to a contingency management intervention (Sheidow et al., 2006). A second study (Henggeler et al., 2007) is examining the determinants of mental health and substance abuse practitioners' interest in and implementation of contingency management techniques. In a third study, the multiple determinants of MST treatment fidelity are being evaluated across more than 40 research sites (e.g., Schoenwald et al., 2003). Together, findings from this research should provide valuable lessons supporting the effective transport and implementation of evidence-based treatments for adolescent substance abuse.

CONCLUSION

Several randomized clinical trials have shown that MST is an effective treatment of adolescent substance use, abuse, and dependence. Youths in MST treatment conditions, in comparison with counterparts receiving alternative services, have demonstrated reduced substance use, decreased criminal activity, improved mental health symptoms, increased school attendance, and reduced rates of out-of-home placement. Moreover, in separate studies, MST has been shown to reduce drug use and drug related crimes at 4- and 14-year follow-ups. In light of these favorable outcomes, research attention has begun to focus on testing strategies for further enhancing the effectiveness of MST in treating substance abuse and on determining the conditions needed for the effective transport of MST and other evidence-based treatments. Hopefully, this research will enhance MST outcomes and inform the transport of other evidence-based practices to community settings.

REFERENCES

Azrin, N. H., Donohue, B., Teichner, G. A., Crum, T., Howell, J., & DeCato, L. A. (2001). A controlled evaluation and description of individual-cognitive problem solving and family-behavior therapies in dually-diagnosed conduct-disordered and substance-dependent youth. *Journal of Child & Adolescent Substance Abuse, 11*, 1-43.

Borduin, C. M., Henggeler, S. W., Blaske, D. M., & Stein, R. J. (1990). Multisystemic treatment of adolescent sexual offenders. *International Journal of Offender Therapy & Comparative Criminology, 34*, 105-113.

Borduin, C. M., Mann, B. J., Cone, L. T., Henggeler, S. W., Fucci, B. R., Blaske, D. M. et al. (1995). Multisystemic treatment of serious juvenile offenders: Long-term prevention of criminality and violence. *Journal of Consulting & Clinical Psychology, 63*, 569-578.

Borduin, C. M., & Schaeffer, C. M. (2001). Multisystemic treatment of juvenile sexual offenders: A progress report. *Journal of Psychology & Human Sexuality, 13*, 25-42.

Bronfenbrenner, U. (1979). *The ecology of human development: Experiments by nature and design.* Cambridge, MA: Harvard University Press.

Brown, T. L., Henggeler, S. W., Schoenwald, S. K., Brondino, M. J., & Pickrel, S. G. (1999). Multisystemic treatment of substance abusing and dependent juvenile delinquents: Effects on school attendance at posttreatment and 6-month follow-up. *Children's Services: Social Policy, Research, & Practice, 2*, 81-93.

Budney, A. J., & Higgins, S. T. (1998). *A community reinforcement plus vouchers approach: Treating cocaine addiction* (NIH Publication No. 98-4309). Rockville, MD: U.S. Department of Health and Human Services, National Institutes of Health, National Institute on Drug Abuse.

Burns, B. J., Hoagwood, K., & Mrazek, P. J. (1999). Effective treatment for mental disorders in children and adolescents. *Clinical Child & Family Psychology Review, 2*, 199-254.

Center for Substance Abuse Prevention. (2001). *Exemplary substance abuse prevention programs award ceremony*. Washington, DC: Substance Abuse and Mental Health Services Administration, Author.

Crowley, T. J., Mikulich, S. K., MacDonald, M., Young, S. E., & Zerbe, G. O. (1998). Substance-dependent, conduct-disordered adolescent males: Severity of diagnosis predicts 2-year outcome. *Drug & Alcohol Dependence, 49*, 225-237.

Curtis, N. M., Ronan, K. R., & Borduin, C. M. (2004). Multisystemic Treatment: A meta-analysis of outcome studies. *Journal of Family Psychology, 18*, 411-419.

Elliott, D. S. (Ed.) (1998). *Blueprints for violence prevention*. Boulder, CO: University of Colorado, Center for the Study and Prevention of Violence, Blueprints Publications.

Farrington, D. P., & Welsh, B. C. (1999). Delinquency prevention using family-based interventions. *Children & Society, 13*, 287-303.

Haley, J. (1987). *Problem-solving therapy (2nd ed.)*. San Francisco, CA: Jossey-Bass.

Hawkins, J. D., Herrenkohl, T., Farrington, D. P., Brewer, D., Catalano, R. F., & Harachi, T. W. (1998). A review of predictors of youth violence. In R. Loeber & D. P. Farrington (Eds.), *Serious & violent juvenile offenders: Risk factors and successful interventions*. (pp. 106-146). Thousand Oaks, CA: Sage Publications.

Henggeler, S. W., Borduin, C. M., Melton, G. B., Mann, B. J., Smith, L., Hall, J. A. et al. (1991). Effects of multisystemic therapy on drug use and abuse in serious juvenile offenders: A progress report from two outcome studies. *Family Dynamics of Addiction Quarterly, 1*, 40-51.

Henggeler, S. W., Chapman, J. E., Rowland, M. D., Halliday-Boykins, C. A., Randall, J., Shackelford, J. et al. (2007). If you build it, they will come: Statewide practitioner interest in CM youths. *Journal of Substance Abuse Treatment*.

Henggeler, S. W., Clingempeel, W. G., Brondino, M. J., & Pickrel, S. G. (2002). Four-year follow-up of multisystemic therapy with substance-abusing and substance-dependent juvenile offenders. *Journal of the American Academy of Child & Adolescent Psychiatry, 41*, 868-874.

Henggeler, S. W., Halliday-Boykins, C. A., Cunningham, P. B., Randall, J., Shapiro, S. B., & Chapman, J. E. (2006). Juvenile drug court: Enhancing outcomes by integrating evidence-based treatments. *Journal of Consulting & Clinical Psychology, 74*.

Henggeler, S. W., Melton, G. B., Brondino, M. J., Scherer, D. G., & Hanley, J. H. (1997). Multisystemic therapy with violent and chronic juvenile offenders and their families: The role of treatment fidelity in successful dissemination. *Journal of Consulting & Clinical Psychology, 65*, 821-833.

Henggeler, S. W., Melton, G. B., & Smith, L. A. (1992). Family preservation using multisystemic therapy: An effective alternative to incarcerating serious juvenile offenders. *Journal of Consulting & Clinical Psychology, 60*, 953-961.

Henggeler, S. W., Pickrel, S. G., & Brondino, M. J. (1999). Multisystemic treatment of substance abusing and dependent delinquents: Outcomes, treatment fidelity, and transportability. *Mental Health Services Research, 1*, 171-184.

Henggeler, S. W., Pickrel, S. G., Brondino, M. J., & Crouch, J. L. (1996). Eliminating (almost) treatment dropout of substance abusing or dependent delinquents through home-based multisystemic therapy. *American Journal of Psychiatry, 153*, 427-428.

Henggeler, S. W., Rodick, J. D., Borduin, C. M., Hanson, C. L., Watson, S. M., & Urey, J. R. (1986). Multisystemic treatment of juvenile offenders: Effects on adolescent behavior and family interaction. *Developmental Psychology, 22*, 132-141.

Henggeler, S. W., & Schoenwald, S. K. (1998). *The MST supervisory manual: Promoting quality assurance at the clinical level.* Charleston, SC: MST Services.

Henggeler, S. W., Schoenwald, S. K., Borduin, C. M., Rowland, M. D., & Cunningham, P. B. (1998). *Multisystemic treatment of antisocial behavior in children and adolescents.* New York: Guilford Press.

Henggeler, S. W., Schoenwald, S. K., Rowland, M. D., & Cunningham, P. B. (2002). *Serious emotional disturbance in children and adolescents: Multisystemic therapy.* New York: Guilford Press.

Huey, S. J., Jr., Henggeler, S. W., Brondino, M. J., & Pickrel, S. G. (2000). Mechanisms of change in multisystemic therapy: Reducing delinquent behavior through therapist adherence and improved family and peer functioning. *Journal of Consulting & Clinical Psychology, 68*, 451-467.

Huizinga, D., Loeber, R., & Thornberry, T. P. (1994). *Urban delinquency and substance abuse: Initial findings.* Washington, DC: Office of Juvenile Justice and Delinquency Prevention, U.S. Department of Justice.

Jones, H. E., Wong, C. J., Tuten, M., & Stitzer, M. L. (2005). Reinforcement-based therapy: 12-month evaluation of an outpatient drug-free treatment for heroin abusers. *Drug and Alcohol Dependence, 79*, 119-128.

Kazdin, A. E., & Weisz, J. R. (1998). Identifying and developing empirically supported child and adolescent treatments. *Journal of Consulting & Clinical Psychology, 66*, 19-36.

Kendall, P. C., & Braswell, L. (1993). *Cognitive-behavioral therapy for impulsive children, 2nd Edition.* New York: Guilford Press.

King, R. D., Gaines, L. S., Lambert, E. W., Summerfelt, W. T., & Bickman, L. (2000). The co-occurrence of psychiatric substance use diagnoses in adolescents in different service systems: Frequency, recognition, cost, and outcomes. *Journal of Behavioral Health Services & Research, 27*, 417-430.

Mihalic, S., Irwin, K., Elliott, D., Fagan, A., & Hansen, D. (2001). *Blueprints for violence prevention.* Boulder, CO: Center for the Study of Violence Prevention.

Minuchin, S. (1974). *Families & family therapy.* Cambridge, MA: Harvard University Press.

Munger, R. L. (1993). *Changing children's behavior quickly.* Lanham, MD: Madison.

National Clearinghouse on Child Abuse and Neglect Information. (2003). *Substance abuse and child maltreatment.* Washington, DC: Department of Health and Human Services, Administration for Children and Families.

National Institute on Drug Abuse. (1999). *Principles of drug addiction treatment: A research-based guide* (NIH Publication No. 99-4180). Rockville, MD: U.S. Department of Health and Human Services, National Institutes of Health, Author.

Office of Applied Studies. (2000). National survey of substance abuse treatment services (N-SSATS).

Ogden, T., & Halliday-Boykins, C. A. (2004). Multisystemic treatment of antisocial adolescents in Norway: Replication of clinical outcomes outside of the US. *Child and Adolescent Mental Health, 9,* 77-83.

Petry, N. M. (2000). A comprehensive guide to the application of contingency management procedures in clinical settings. *Drug & Alcohol Dependence, 58,* 9-25.

President's New Freedom Commission on Mental Health. (2003). *Achieving the Promise: Transforming Mental Health Care in America.*

Schaeffer, C. M., & Borduin, C. M. (2005). Long-term follow-up to a randomized clinical trial of multisystemic therapy with serious and violent juvenile offenders. *Journal of Consulting and Clinical Psychology, 73,* 445-453.

Schaeffer, C. M., Saldana, L., Rowland, M. D., Henggeler, S. W., & Swenson, C. C. (in press). New initiatives in improving youth and family outcomes by importing evidence-based practices. *Journal of Child & Adolescent Substance Abuse.*

Schoenwald, S. K. (1998). *Multisystemic therapy consultation guidelines.* Charleston, SC: MST Institute.

Schoenwald, S. K., Sheidow, A. J., Letourneau, E. J., & Liao, J. G. (2003). Transportability of evidence-based treatments: Evidence for multi-level influences. *Mental Health Services Research, 5,* 223-239.

Schoenwald, S. K., Ward, D. M., Henggeler, S. W., Pickrel, S. G., & Patel, H. (1996). Multisystemic therapy treatment of substance abusing or dependent adolescent offenders: Costs of reducing incarceration, inpatient, and residential placement. *Journal of Child & Family Studies, 5,* 431-444.

Sheidow, A. J., Henggeler, S. W., Cunningham, P. B., Donohue, B. C., Ford, J. D., & Shapiro, S. B. (2006). Transporting contingency management for youth treated with Multisystemic Therapy. In S. K. Schoenwald (Chair), *Key findings in the transport and implementation of evidence-based treatments to community settings.* Symposium conducted at the annual Joint Meeting on Adolescent Treatment Effectiveness, Baltimore, MD.

Sheidow, A. J., Molen, L. A., Navas-Murphy, L., & Chapman, J. E. (2007). Stage I research evaluating an outpatient treatment for co-occurring substance use & internalizing problems. In A. J. Sheidow (Chair), *Co-occurring substance use and mental health problems: Recent findings from transportability and clinical research.* Symposium to be conducted at the annual Joint Meeting on Adolescent Treatment Effectiveness, Washington, DC.

Stanton, M. D., & Shadish, W. R. (1997). Outcome, attrition, and family-couples treatment for drug abuse: A meta-analysis and review of the controlled, comparative studies. *Psychological Bulletin, 122,* 170-191.

Stark, M. J. (1992). Dropping out of substance abuse treatment: A clinically oriented review. *Clinical Psychology Review, 12,* 93-116.

Substance Abuse and Mental Health Services Administration. (2007). *SAMHSA model programs: Multisystemic therapy*. Rockville, MD: U.S. Department of Health and Human Services, Author.

Swenson, C. C., Henggeler, S. W., Taylor, I. S., & Addison, O. W. (2005). *Multisystemic therapy and neighborhood partnerships: Reducing adolescent violence and substance abuse*. New York: Guilford Press.

Swenson, C. C., Saldana, L., Joyner, C. D., Caldwell, E., Henggeler, S. W., & Rowland, M. D. (2005). *Multisystemic Therapy for child abuse and neglect*. Charleston: Medical University of South Carolina, Family Services Research Center.

Timmons-Mitchell, J., Bender, M. B., Kishna, M. A., & Mitchell, C. C. (2006). An independent effectiveness trial of Multisystemic Therapy with juvenile justice youth. *Journal of Clinical Child and Adolescent Psychology, 35*, 227-236.

U.S. Public Health Service. (1999). *Mental health: A report of the Surgeon General*. Rockville, MD: U.S. Department of Health and Human Services, National Institutes of Health, National Institute of Mental Health.

U.S. Public Health Service. (2001). *Youth violence: A report of the Surgeon General*. Washington, DC: Author.

von Bertalanffy, L. (1968). *General system theory: Foundations, development, applications*. New York: Braziller.

Weinberg, N. Z., Rahdert, E., Colliver, J. D., & Glantz, M. D. (1998). Adolescent substance abuse: A review of the past 10 years. *Journal of the American Academy of Child & Adolescent Psychiatry, 37*, 252-261.

doi:10.1300/J020v26n01_07

Invitational Intervention:
The ARISE Model
for Engaging Reluctant Alcohol
and Other Drug Abusers in Treatment

Judith Landau, MD
James Garrett, CSW

SUMMARY. Families are an untapped resource in motivating resistant alcohol dependent and other drug addicted individuals to enter treatment. Contrary to popular belief, families maintain a disproportionately close connectedness with their addicted loved ones. In this article, the authors present the underlying functional components of this connectedness, and describe the process called Family Motivation to Change for mobilizing family and friends to form an Intervention Network for the express

---

Judith Landau and James Garrett are affiliated with Linking Human Systems™ in Boulder, CO.

Address correspondence to: Judith Landau, Linking Human Systems, LLC, 964 Grant Place, Boulder, CO 80302 (E-mail: JLandau@LinkingHumanSystems.com. or Web: LinkingHumanSystems.com).

The authors would like to express thanks to an anonymous reviewer for helpful comments on an earlier draft of this paper.

The empirical study from which this work has been further developed was supported in major part by the National Institute on Drug Abuse (NIDA–grant No. RO1 DA09402), National Institutes of Health.

[Haworth co-indexing entry note]: "Invitational Intervention: The ARISE Model for Engaging Reluctant Alcohol and Other Drug Abusers in Treatment." Landau, Judith, and James Garrett. Co-published simultaneously in *Alcoholism Treatment Quarterly* (The Haworth Press) Vol. 26, No. 1/2, 2008, pp. 147-168; and: *Family Intervention in Substance Abuse: Current Best Practices* (ed: Oliver J. Morgan, and Cheryl H. Litzke) The Haworth Press, 2008, pp. 147-168. Single or multiple copies of this article are available for a fee from The Haworth Document Delivery Service [1-800-HAWORTH, 9:00 a.m. - 5:00 p.m. (EST). E-mail address: docdelivery@haworthpress.com].

purpose of getting a resistant addicted loved one into treatment. This is the core of ARISE as **A R**elational **I**ntervention **S**equence for **E**ngagement. ARISE uses an Invitational Intervention method, with the family conducting most of the Intervention, thus minimizing the clinician's expenditure of time and cost. doi:10.1300/J020v26n01_08 *[Article copies available for a fee from The Haworth Document Delivery Service: 1-800-HAWORTH. E-mail address: <docdelivery@haworthpress.com> Website: <http://www.HaworthPress.com> © 2008 by The Haworth Press. All rights reserved.]*

KEYWORDS. ARISE, treatment engagement, Invitational Intervention, alcoholism in the family, alcohol-other drug abuse, family motivation, motivation to change, concerned other

INTRODUCTION

The major problem confronting the field of addiction is the low rate at which alcoholics and other substance abusers enter treatment. In fact, the majority, less than 10%, ever does so (Frances, Miller, & Galanter, 1989; Nathan, 1990; Kessler et al., 1994). These statistics are found not only in the United States, but also elsewhere around the world. This low rate of treatment entry causes difficulties for members of the family and extended support system because each person is affected by the disease and its accompanying problems.

For instance, a busy primary care physician or nurse practitioner might dread the appearance of a particular patient in the examining room, predicting that s/he is likely to have developed yet another psychosomatic symptom, or be requesting days off work to deal with some minor illness or infection. Many primary care providers have come to realize that the underlying problem rendering the person particularly vulnerable is most likely to be stress. Unfortunately, fewer are likely to realize that there is a high probability that the patient's spouse is struggling with chronic addiction, and that the patient in the office is exhibiting relational symptoms of the disease.

This paper describes ARISE (A Relational Intervention Sequence for Engagement), a manual-driven relational intervention designed to guide family members to get a resistant substance abuser into treatment. It draws on the connectedness, interest and commitment of other concerned members of the extended family and support system to motivate the alcoholic or substance abuser to enter treatment. The ARISE Interventionist collaborates, or "partners," with extended families and their support networks, mobilizing them to act as motivational enhancers to get addicted individuals into treatment.

OVERVIEW OF INTERVENTION

Those familiar with family therapy understand "intervention" to describe a clinical technique used by a therapist to accomplish a clinical goal. Those familiar with addiction treatment understand "Intervention" to mean a specific technique designed to assist families and significant others to induce an alcohol dependent or addicted individual to enter treatment. This paper will focus on the latter use of the word "Intervention," with a capital "I" denoting the technique designed to get resistant alcohol dependent or addicted individuals into treatment.

Informal Interventions

The basic idea behind any intervention is a desire by family, friends, clergy, colleagues, neighbors, care providers, employers, and other members of the support network to take an active role in assisting another person to change unacceptable behavior. The idea of intervention has been around as long as one person has tried to influence the behavior of another. Everyone has done some form of intervention with others. Perhaps one has tried to help a friend who is chronically late for work get to work on time; prompted someone who was erratic about taking prescriptions to take medication on a regular basis; tried to get a loved one to stop smoking cigarettes; or struggled to persuade a colleague to start an exercise program to help with weight loss. These are examples of simple interventions where one person is working to motivate another to change a behavior. This type of intervention is a frequent, daily occurrence. It is usually informal, focused on one objective, and works through applying the power of the emotional connection in personal relationships towards motivating change.

Substance Abuse Interventions

The toll of untreated addiction can be seen in many direct and indirect costs to society, including: health care, criminal justice, child welfare, employment, family/marital functioning and mental health. For instance, the alcohol dependent or addicted individual uses 4 times the health care dollars used by non-addicted individuals. Concurrently, National Institute on Drug Abuse (NIDA) studies show that of the 2 million admissions per year into addiction treatment facilities, 75% of drug addicts and alcoholics credit their families as the major reason for their getting into treatment (McCrady, 2006): Families are powerful motivators for alcohol dependent and addicted individuals to get treatment.

Combining these two factors, the cost of addiction and the leverage of families, Vernon Johnson, some 35 years ago, popularized the first Intervention method with his publication, *I'll Quit Tomorrow* (Johnson, 1973). The method was designed to capitalize on the family's interest in getting their resistant alcoholic into treatment. The Johnson Intervention method remained the primary method used until fairly recently. During the past 15 years, several new Intervention methods have developed including: Unilateral Intervention (Thomas & Ager, 1993); Community Reinforcement and Family Training (CRAFT) (Miller & Myers, 1996); A Relational Intervention Sequence for Engagement (ARISE) (Garrett et al., 1997, 1998, 1999; Landau et al., 2000, 2004); Structural Strategic Intervention With Adolescents (Szapocznik et al., 1988) and the (currently unpublished) Systemic Intervention Model (Raiter & Toll, 2006; Maher, 2006).

The common thread through the above-mentioned Intervention methods is the focus on getting a resistant addicted individual into treatment. Some of the methods use a unilateral approach (Unilateral Intervention and CRAFT) and the others employ a systemic approach (Johnson Intervention, Systemic Intervention and ARISE). Of the systemic methods only ARISE uses an Invitational Intervention method. The other systemic methods utilize a surprise approach to reaching the addicted individual.

WHY AN INVITATION?

The historical dilemma, when doing an Intervention, has been how to get the alcohol dependent or addicted individual to participate in a session to discuss an alcohol/drug problem that the individual does not believe exists. The earlier systemic methods thought it best to "surprise" the individual and that way assure having a "captive" audience for the Intervention meeting. The idea of inviting an alcohol dependent or addicted individual to attend a meeting about a problem s/he believes does not exist, would seem an inevitable prescription for failure. Alternatively, not offering the invitation, and proceeding to have a secret meeting without the individual, or springing a surprise meeting on him or her, would almost definitely result in a defiant, rebellious response. The old adage applies, "Tell me what to do and I will do the exact opposite."

The question of why to invite an addicted individual to attend a meeting where his/her problem of alcohol and drug use will be discussed is based on the principles of family connectedness and the dynamics of Family Motivation to Change (Garrett & Landau, 2006). In the late 1980's the authors researched this question of invitation thoroughly. They did a retrospective analysis of some 350 individuals admitted to an Intensive Outpatient Program (IOP) for addiction treatment. These individuals met three evenings each week for sixteen weeks. The study sample was divided according to three significant dynamics that had motivated the addicted individual to start treatment: self-referral, court mandate, and Johnson Intervention (Loneck, Garrett, & Banks, 1996a; 1996 b).

This retrospective analysis examined the rates of treatment completion and relapse during the course of treatment. The lowest treatment completion rate (40%) was in the self-referred population. The highest completion rate (91%) was in the court-mandated group. The Johnson Intervention group completion rate was 55%. It is interesting to note that the group that on the surface had the best motivation at the start of treatment (self-referred) had the highest treatment dropout rate. The authors further studied the self-referral group in an attempt to under-stand this apparent discrepancy. They found that the high dropout rate was directly related to the lack of a consequence for dropping out. This self-referred group had no one, other than themselves, to be accountable to when deciding to leave treatment. At the other end of the spectrum, the court mandated group had the most immediate consequence for dropping out of treatment and, therefore, the highest treatment completion rate. The Johnson Intervention group started off strong in treatment, but had high rates of dropping out after eight to ten weeks.

The dynamics of relapse may explain the timing of the Johnson Inter-vention group's dropout rate with relapses occurring between the sixth and eighth week of treatment. Dropout rates increased as relapses occurred. During follow-up interviews with the Johnson Intervention group, the authors heard a familiar statement over and over. "At first, I stopped my drug and alcohol use because of the pressure from the Inter-vention, but then I found myself thinking 'I'm not going to be told what to do!' so I started using again."

This finding led the authors to wonder whether the rebellious response and subsequent pattern of relapse noted in the Johnson Intervention group could be avoided by using a method that started with an invitation rather than by surprise or coercion.

Another study by the authors in the 1980s further bolstered their rationale for starting ARISE with an invitational meeting. Data collected from all calls from family members requesting help to get an addicted loved one into treatment revealed that more than eight of every ten families refused to follow through with a Johnson Intervention (the only model being offered at the time). Following this early study, other research has resulted in similar findings. For example, in 1997, Barber and Gilbertson reported that 100% of the women in their Australian study refused to do a Johnson Intervention when it was offered.

Based on these findings, the authors did a qualitative study exploring the barriers to participation in the Johnson Intervention. They interviewed a sample of families who had refused to do a Johnson Intervention. Some of the reasons the families gave are listed below:

- Fear that the highly confrontational aspects of the method would destroy the relationship with the addicted individual and/or chase him away forever;
- Belief that support for the addicted individual was more important than developing harsh consequences;
- Fear that the addicted individual would "go over the edge" if strongly confronted; and
- Skepticism that any method would work, deriving from the family's sense of isolation, confusion and despair from living for a long time with active addiction.

The other aspect, that of connection of the alcohol dependent or addicted individual to his/her family of origin is well documented (Stanton & Shadish, 1997). In fact, contrary to the common perception in the field, alcoholics care about their families and their families care about them. They remain very closely connected; in fact, more closely connected than the general population. Averaging several studies, it appears that 9% of non-addicts tend to call their families daily while addicted persons maintain daily contact with their families at a rate of approximately 57% in the US, 62% in England, 80% in Thailand and Italy, and 67% in Puerto Rico (Perzel & Lamon, 1979; Vaillant, 1995). One might ask, where did this connectedness originate and how does it relate to addiction?

The authors have found that addictive symptoms originate in families as an attempt at adaptive behavior to cope with transitional conflict arising from migration, rapid or unpredictable transitions, traumatic loss, and unresolved grief (Landau, 2005; Garrett & Landau, 2006; Landau & Garrett, 2006). Other symptomatic behaviors include: depression and suicidality, violence, post-traumatic stress, and risk-taking behaviors, including those that can lead to HIV/AIDS (Landau, 2005; Landau & Saul, 2004). For example, within one year after September 11th, 2001, there was a 31% increase in the rate of substance abuse and addiction in New York City and its immediate surroundings, approximating the addiction statistics of uprooted persons around the world (Johnson, Richter, McClellan, & Kleber, 2002). At times of overwhelming grief, families find ways of compensating and staying close together to avoid further loss, often without conscious intent.

Frequently, one member of the family will begin to use alcohol or other substances, or exhibit other symptoms that serve the dual purpose of drawing the family's attention away from the grief and holding the family together to deal with the problems arising from the new problem behavior or symptoms. The result is that the family is unable to process their current transitions, remaining locked in the transitional conflict of the moment. Since this maintains their closeness, the substance use helps to assuage the grief and reduce the pain. When the substance use is reduced, the pain and grief return to the family, reinforcing the need for the problem, increased use, or a relapse from recovery results. The addiction cycle is set. It has proven effective in assuaging grief and maintaining family connectedness to prevent further loss.

Because it is successful in its purpose, the pattern of substance use, relief of grief, and relapse if the grief occurs when recovery begins, is often transmitted across generations. This continues until the family grieving is resolved, the substance use or abuse has become redundant, and healing of the family and the substance abuser can occur (Landau, 1979, 1981; Landau & Stanton, 1990; Landau, Garrett et al., 2000; Landau, 2004a, 2004b). This pattern is totally subconscious. If the grieving is not resolved within a couple of generations, it is likely to spread laterally on the family genogram as well as vertically down the generations. Once the grieving is done, generally 3 to 5 generations later if no therapeutic intervention has occurred, another member of the family moves into recovery, often spontaneously.

The authors have termed this survival drive of the family "Family Motivation to Change" (Garrett & Landau, 2006). The family does not have to wait until the grieving is done. Intervention is possible and can capitalize on the healing energy of the family to prevent generations of addiction and grief. The motivation of family members to get an addicted loved one into treatment occurs when one or more individuals agree to take action to stop the alcohol or drug use from taking its progressive toll and distracting the family from functioning in a more healthy manner. Family Motivation to Change can best be understood as the combined forces operating within a family that guide it first towards maintaining survival in the face of serious threat, or following major or unpredictable loss and unresolved grief. Secondly, the same Family Motivation to Change guides the family towards health and sustained functioning when threat is removed.

Exploring what happened to families during major disaster, traumatic or unexpected loss, or multiple losses allowed the authors to take a step back into the grief that initiated the problem of addiction (Garrett & Landau, 2006). The authors discovered that the force that drives a family towards health is the same force that drove them to the initial adaptive behavior described above, where a family member becomes addicted in an attempt to keep the family close and to prevent them from feeling the pain of intense loss and sorrow. Eventually, the focus on the problems caused by the individual's alcoholism or drug addiction slows the process of successfully completing normal family life cycle transitions until the grief is resolved.

Once this has happened, the driving force of health and healing, "Family Motivation to Change," pushes, frees, or allows a member of the family, a natural change agent or Family Link to lead the family out of grief and addiction and into health and recovery (Landau, 1979, 1982; Landau-Stanton & Clements, 1993; Landau, 2004a).

Understanding the dynamics related to family connectedness and Family Motivation to Change resulted in the development of an Intervention method that built on the respect and long-term commitment of family members to maintain relationships with one another. The result was the development of a three-level Intervention method that started with an invitation.

ARISE Overview

ARISE is rooted in concepts and methods developed both from addiction theory and from family and systems theory particularly social network therapy (Speck & Attneave, 1973), Transitional Family Therapy (Seaburn, Horwitz, & Landau, 1995) and the network approach to substance abuse treatment (Galanter, 1993). Although ARISE draws heavily from theories used in family and systems therapy, it is a pre-treatment engagement technique and is not therapy. Therefore, professionals using ARISE are not practicing therapy, but are solely focused on getting the addicted individual into treatment and the family as a whole into recovery.

ARISE is manual-driven, and has been formally investigated (Landau et al., 2004).[1] The ARISE method evolved during the late 1970's and was formalized in the mid-1980s. As mentioned earlier, its development was driven by families' refusing to use the Johnson Intervention combined with the integration of systems theory into addictions treatment. Rather than viewing the families as being "wrong" or "uncaring" for not following through on the Intervention method offered, the authors built on their knowledge of family systems, trust in family competence, strength and resilience, and their prior experience of family members' success in getting substance abusers into treatment (Landau & Garrett, 2006). ARISE evolved as a user-friendly and cost-effective intervention method.

Most families who were initially not interested in participating in an Intervention because of their preconceived notions or prior conceptions, became interested and willing to use the ARISE method because of the openness and lack of confrontation. Families learn that ARISE focuses attention not only on treatment engagement of the individual substance abuser, but on long-term intergenerational family well-being and recovery. They also feel hopeful for the future, once they realize that their ongoing relationship with their alcohol dependent or addicted member will be honored and protected.

The following summarizes the 3 Levels of ARISE: *Level 1* uses motivational techniques designed specifically for telephone coaching, but they can also be applied to face-to-face sessions. We help the "First Caller" or "Concerned Other" establish a basis of hope, identify whom to invite to the initial Intervention meeting, design a strategy to mobilize the support group, teach techniques to successfully invite the alcohol dependent or addicted individual to the first meeting, suggest a recovery message and get a commitment from all invited individuals to attend the initial meeting regardless of whether or not the alcoholic attends. *Level 2* follows if treatment does not start during Level 1. Typically, in Level 2, between two to five face-to-face sessions are held, with or without the alcohol dependent or addicted individual present, to mobilize the Intervention Network in developing motivational strategies to attain the goal of treatment engagement. Very few families (less than 2%) need to proceed to Level 3. In *Level 3*, family and friends set limits and consequences for the alcohol dependent or addicted individual in a loving and supportive way. By the time the Intervention Network gets to this point, the alcohol dependent or addicted individual has been given and has refused many opportunities to enter treatment. Because the alcohol dependent or addicted individual has been invited to each of the Intervention Network meetings in Level 1 and Level 2, this final limit setting approach is a natural consequence and does not come as a surprise. The Intervention Network commits to supporting each other in the implementation of the agreed upon consequences.

CASE EXAMPLES AT EACH OF THE THREE LEVELS

Level 1 Case

The First Caller was a mother, Jan, who was concerned about the alcohol and cocaine use of her 29-year-old son, Jude. Jan had learned earlier in the week from her son's wife Margaret that Jude had spent close to $6,500 of an inheritance over the previous three months. The concern was that the money had been spent secretly and that Margaret could not identify anything that had been bought. During the First Call, Jan related that her son had a long-standing problem with drinking, but she did not know of any use of cocaine or other drugs.

A section of the First Call Worksheet calls for constructing a preliminary genogram. The purpose of this is to get a family history, list individuals who might be willing to attend the First Meeting and/or be of support during the Invitational Intervention process, and to identify themes and patterns that could be useful in developing the Recovery Message. The Recovery Message is an essential and central component of the invitation that is conveyed to the alcohol dependent or addicted individual.

The genogram revealed that Jude's father, Mark, had been a "dry alcoholic" for the past 15 years. Mark stopped drinking on his own after a series of violent domestic episodes while he was intoxicated. These incidents had resulted in Jan's divorcing him. Jude and Margaret had been married for 4 years and had a 2-year-old daughter, Samantha. It was also noted that both of Jude's grandfathers were alcoholic. His fraternal grandfather had also stopped drinking later in life and had attended AA meetings for a period of time. Jude's fraternal grandfather had passed away approximately 3 months before the First Call, and Jan stated that her son had spent nearly every day with his grandfather in the nursing home for the two months prior to his death.

When asked who might be willing to attend the First Meeting, Jan constructed the following list: herself (mother); Margaret (wife); Mark (father); Pat (sister); Margaret's parents; and two of Jude's friends with whom he drank and used drugs. When discussing this list in more detail it was decided that it would be best not to invite Margaret's parents to the first meeting, due to recent hostility between them and Jude. It was also decided not to invite the two friends because of concerns about whether they would support Jude's entry into treatment.

One of the key issues in reducing the size of the Intervention Network was that Jan and her ex-husband, Mark, had not been in the same room together since their divorce. Jan thought it would be more productive and provide a better forum for openness if the initial group was smaller, comprising only immediate family who knew the history of violence. She also revealed, "for years after the divorce Jude would sleep in the hallway outside my door because he thought he had to protect me." Jude had no history of violence.

When deciding when and where to meet, it was decided to give Jude a choice of either meeting at his home, his mother's home, or in the Interventionist's office. The Recovery Message that would be the central component of the invitation was "We know you do not want your daughter to grow up scared and insecure like you did. Let's not let these problems carry over into the next generation."

Jan approached her son two days before the date of the First Meeting and shared with him her concerns, her contact with the ARISE Interventionist, the date and time for the First Meeting, and who was going to attend. She asked where he would prefer the First Meeting to take place and conveyed the Recovery Message. She ended the invitation by letting Jude know that the Intervention Network would be meeting regardless of whether or not he decided to attend.

Jude was 45 minutes late for the First Meeting. The initial time without him was spent with the family discussing the family's history of alcoholism, their inter-generational history of violence, and Jan and Mark's courage and love in being prepared to be in the same room together for the shared goal of getting their son into treatment and breaking the cycle of alcoholism in the family.

When Jude came into the First Meeting, he sat down and looked at his parents and stated, "I'll bet you thought I wasn't coming. I didn't come on time on purpose. I knew you had things to discuss on your own without me." Both parents shared what had been discussed and stated the purpose of the meeting. Jude was asked to listen while each person shared with him his or her concerns. Each person shared what s/he knew of his alcohol and drug use and requested that he get help.

After listening to them, Jude was given an opportunity to respond. He admitted to his problem with alcohol and cocaine. He talked about how his cocaine use escalated after his grandfather had died, and how he had been having recurrent thoughts of his own death since losing his grandfather. The group supported him, validating how each of them was also having a difficult time with the grandfather's death. Jude agreed to check into a local hospital detox unit the next day and the family agreed to meet again in the detox unit to discuss the next level of care needed.

Level 2 Case

The First Caller was the mother of 16-year-old Angela, who had been sexually assaulted at the age of 14 by a 28-year-old man who had plied her with drink and taken advantage of her once she was intoxicated. Angela had been through an extremely painful unsuccessful court case. Despite the statutory rape, her rapist had been found not guilty because the emergency room physician had failed to take the necessary samples at the time of her medical examination. Angela's mother had called to request help because Angela was drinking heavily and using marijuana on a daily basis. She was also failing almost every class in school, playing truant with friends, and whenever her parents tried to discipline her, she would run away, once even running through traffic on a busy highway, narrowly escaping death. During the previous 3 months, Angela had been involved in 4 car accidents of escalating seriousness. Her parents felt that she was depressed and were reluctant to discipline her too strictly in case that put even more pressure on her and drove her further into depression or suicidality. They were beside themselves, but felt helpless to change the situation.

Angela attended all 3 Level I First Call meetings, along with her parents and all 3 of her siblings, but she refused to consider treatment for her addiction and depression. Whenever action was mentioned, she would burst into floods of tears alternating with fury at her father, stating, "You're one to talk! You always drink when you're upset! Why don't you go for treatment?" Her father, after some intense family conflict, agreed to stop drinking if that would help Angela get into treatment and get better. The genogram revealed that Angela's maternal grandmother, with whom she had been very close, had died recently.

It became clear that both Angela and her mother were still grieving. The parents had lost their first child at 18 months from a congenital illness. This loss was followed by Angela's mother being diagnosed with malignant melanoma, and years after treatment she now suffered from Chronic Fatigue Syndrome. Angela and the other siblings felt that they had been forced to raise themselves as father buried himself in his workaholism and mother stayed in her bed.

Once the grief had been identified, and the family was able to work through their extensive losses, it became apparent why the parents were terrified of disciplining Angela. They were anxious about not suffering yet another loss.

After 3 Level I meetings, it was clear that the system needed to be expanded, and friends and extended family members were invited to bring their "Strength in Numbers" at Level II. With some clear consequences set for her behavior, and the other members of the support system not falling for Angela's threats, the parents became visibly stronger and were able to insist that she go into an alternative school system with intensive addiction programming. Clear parameters were set for Angela's completing the required program, and she agreed to the conditions with clear relief that safe boundaries were being set. She did extremely well in the program, and was able to graduate from high school with honors and attend the college of her choice. In fact, she chose to attend a college with a dry campus, and is doing extremely well in academics and her social life.

Level 3 Case

The First Caller was the step-grandmother, Sara, who called regarding the problems her 48-year-old step-granddaughter, Julie, was having with alcohol. The problem that prompted the First Call was a school issue that surfaced with Jean, Julie's 17-year-old daughter, and the lack of follow through with a college application.

The participants in the First meeting were: Sara (step grandmother), Frank (father), Jean (17-year-old daughter), Pam (16-year-old daughter), Peggy (friend), and Molly (friend). Sara did the invitation and used the following Recovery Message as part of the inviting: "We know how unhappy you have been over the past few years. You have not been the same since your mother died 10 years ago. Your children need their mother, just like you needed your's. We know how much pain you must be in." Julie did come to the First Meeting and minimized her drinking. She was not willing to enter treatment, but agreed to "cut down" on her drinking. The Intervention Network agreed to continue meeting because they did not agree with Julie's decision and did not think she would be successful at reducing her drinking.

The Intervention Network held 3 additional meetings in the subsequent 5 weeks after the First Meeting. Julie was invited to each of these meetings. She attended the second of the three meetings.

She reported in that meeting about how "successful" she had been at cutting down her drinking. "I have been able to only drink one or two drinks a night and I don't even drink every night anymore." Her reporting of her drinking was contradicted by what others in the Intervention Network had observed. One of her friends, Peggy, reported, "You could barely talk last Saturday night when I stopped over. You had a lot more than one or two drinks." Her father, Frank, shared how he could identify with her minimizing, "Before I went into AA and stopped my drinking I lied about how much and how often I drank. I went to AA meetings and drank before going and shared with the AA group how well I was doing not drinking." Julie refused to enter treatment.

In the 3rd Intervention Network meeting (in Level 2) the group shared growing concerns about Julie and how her drinking had continued to be a problem. The group was concerned because Julie told Molly that "I will never go to another one of those meetings again. I don't have a drinking problem and you are being brainwashed by the rest of the group." Various options were discussed and the Intervention Network agreed to go to a Level 3 session where a consequence would be introduced if Julie did not enter treatment.

Julie was again invited to the Level 3 session with the agreement that this would be the last meeting the group would invite her to attend. She agreed to come.

The start of the Level 3 ARISE Intervention meeting is similar to the First Meeting, where the alcohol dependent or addicted individual is asked to listen to the concerns of each person and then respond at the end.

The group members shared their concerns with each statement ending with a request that Julie get into treatment. Julie's father, Frank, was the last to speak. He was chosen last because he was to introduce the consequence. In this case the consequence was that, if Julie did not enter treatment, her children would be leaving their home and would be living with their grandparents until the time that Julie was stable in an alcoholism recovery program. Julie was shocked by the consequence, tried to single her daughters out to convince them not to leave, and expressed anger over the "threat of taking my children away from me."

Her two friends were able to calmly share the information about the Intervention Network meetings that she had previously been invited to attend and how her plan to reduce her drinking had not worked. The friends were able to tell Julie how the whole group had made the decision and that the group's commitment to the consequence was firm and non-negotiable. The friends invited her to go to Family Court so a judge could hear the merits of her case, hear the history of the alcohol abuse, hear the summary of the Intervention Network meetings, and then make a decision. Julie argued for another 5 minutes. The group got up to leave, including her daughters, who said, "Mom, we will be in touch from Grandpa's house." Julie began to cry and asked the group to sit back down because she could not stand to lose her daughters and would enter treatment.

OUTCOME OF THE NIDA ARISE STUDY

ARISE proved successful at helping concerned others to get their resistant loved ones or friends into substance abuse treatment or self-help in 83% of the cases. The 83% level of success was achieved (a) without excluding any cases who asked for help, and (b) with an average of only one session and 1-2 phone calls, totaling 88 minutes of clinician time (median = 75 min., range 5-375). One of the surprising findings was that Invitational Intervention using the ARISE method achieved engagement very rapidly. Fifty percent of engagers entered treatment within one week from the First Call, and 84% within three weeks (Landau & Stanton et al., 2004). One of the reasons that ARISE appears to be so cost-efficient as an engagement method is that the concerned other, family and support network take responsibility for a major proportion of the work, reducing the time and effort spent by the clinician.

The engagement rate did not differ across demographic variables such as age, gender, or race. Nor did it differ across a number of variables such as preferred substance of abuse (cocaine, alcohol, other drug), current level of substance abuse, length of use, or treatment history (inpatient, outpatient). (See Figure 1).

One variable that did reach significance was the extent to which concerned others deemed their addicted individuals to be in need of treatment: The greater the perceived need, the more likely were they and their network to get the addicted individuals engaged in treatment or self-help. Both these variables can be attributed to the concerned others' level of motivation and their frustration at dealing with the addicted

FIGURE 1. Cumulative engagement rates at each stage of ARISE by primary substance abused

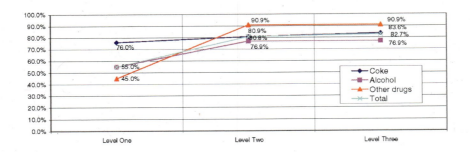

individual's ongoing denial and resistance to treatment. This combination is most likely to lead to the concerned other devoting effort to contacting other network members, convening meetings, and working hard toward getting the substance abuser into treatment.

There was no significant difference among different types of concerned other-addicted individual relationships. However, in line with Meyers et al. (1998) and Miller et al. (1999) finding that parents were more likely to get addicted individuals engaged than spouses, we did find improved results with cases in which at least one parent *was involved as a participant*, whether or not that parent was the actual concerned other (Landau & Stanton et al., 2004). This also matched the research that addicted individuals are closely involved with one or both of their parents. This supports the findings of Meyers et al. (1998), Miller et al. (1999), and Szapocznik et al. (1988) suggesting that parents can be a powerful resource for inducing addicted individuals to seek help.

Engagement at Level I

By the end of Level I, 55% of these cases had been engaged in treatment, requiring only one or two telephone conversations between the clinician and the concerned other and one face-to-face session. We believe this success rate can be attributed to four primary factors:

(1) *Immediacy*. ARISE capitalizes on the timeliness of the concerned other's choosing to call on that particular day. Barriers are minimized and the ARISE Interventionist supports the concerned other's decision to call at that particular time, and translates the situation into reasons

why the concerned other should act now, rather than later. A similar rationale has been employed with the Community Reinforcement Training approach to engagement: the clinician attempts to see the concerned other on the day of the first call (Azrin, 1976; Sisson & Azrin, 1986). Further, the immediacy of a program's response has been shown significantly to increase the rate at which substance abusers, calling in for initial appointments, will actually show up (Festinger, Lamb, Kirby, & Marlowe, 1996; Stasiewicz & Stalker, 1999). In addition, the crisis intervention literature demonstrates the benefit of an immediate response in people faced with crises (Lystad, 1988; Rapaport, 1977).

(2) *Sharing the responsibility* by network support for the concerned other. This starts from the moment of the First Call, when the ARISE Interventionist reassures the concerned other that s/he does not need to handle the situation alone any more, and that help from others breaks the isolation, provides needed support, and dilutes the negative power of the addicted individual who is most likely to "win" in a one-on-one situation. Expanding the system by bringing in additional members of the support network is critical in this process (Landau, 1981; Landau-Stanton & Clements, 1993; Landau et al., 2000).

When the Interventionist works only with the concerned other-addicted individual relationship, he or she is necessarily confined to the dynamics of that relationship. If there is tension or a stalemate, or the relationship has escalated into open conflict, the addicted individual is unlikely to want to hear the demands or wishes of the concerned other. The most stressed dyad is also likely to have the least energy and capacity for change. Sharing the responsibility, and getting the concerned other out of the middle, allows other network members with greater leverage to intervene, bringing additional resources and "strength in numbers" to the Intervention (Landau et al., 2000).

(3) *Instilling Confidence in the Concerned Other.* The clinician starts building confidence by assuring the concerned other that there is a method designed particularly for the situation s/he has just described. This leads to hope where previously there may have been frustration, despair and anger. In addition, the reassurance by the ARISE Interventionist that a Herculean effort may not be required to engage the addicted individual appears less daunting and therefore more achievable. The concerned other is motivated by the knowledge that only the amount of time and effort necessary to effect engagement will be required. Finally, spreading responsibility among other network members both relieves the concerned other of a considerable burden and fortifies the notion that the contributions of these others may increase the

chance that something constructive will result. As Miller et al. (1999) state: there is a "direct message that family members *can* do something to instigate change" (p. 695).

(4) *Respect for the addicted individual* is shown by including him or her in the process from the very start. As mentioned earlier, the Addicted Individual is informed about the First Call and invited to the first ARISE session. The Addicted Individual is also told that, since the discussion will revolve around her or him, s/he may want to attend in order to provide input and have her/his views considered. This alone often succeeds in getting him/her to attend because most people do not like to be talked about without both hearing what is said and having a voice in the discussion. Should s/he not attend that meeting, constant efforts are made to encourage her/him to join the process.

Consequently, there is neither loss of face nor embarrassment if s/he later is persuaded to come in as is likely to happen when the approach has involved secrecy or strong confrontation.

Prevailing Addiction Myths

As with most of the other published engagement studies, these findings challenge the widespread view that addicted individuals must "hit bottom" and be self-motivated to enter treatment. Along these lines Loneck, Garrett, and Banks (1996a, 1996b) found that self-referrals (i.e., those addicted individuals who sought admission on their own after hitting bottom) had the lowest treatment completion rates by comparison with criminal justice referrals and family-type intervention referrals.

Concerned others in the NIDA study often indicated to the ARISE Interventionists that they had tried other agencies without receiving much encouragement. Many mentioned the anger they experienced at being labeled "co-dependent," "controlling," a "victim" or an "enabler," and the helplessness they felt at being told that there was nothing they could do until their loved one "hit bottom." They were relieved and felt supported and encouraged by this Invitational Intervention.

CONCLUSION AND PRACTICAL CLINICAL IMPLICATIONS

Invitational Intervention, and the ARISE protocol, can be applied to a number of non-substance related addictions and dependencies that, in their own way, are as disruptive to individual and family life as substance abuse. These tend to fall into three main categories: (a) other addictions and behavioral compulsions; (b) chronic and/or life-threatening physical or psychiatric disorders, and (c) physical or emotional problems that threaten primary relationships, but are not severe enough to warrant psychiatric referral.

The authors have used Invitational Intervention in the areas listed above. They have not yet done empirical studies, but on an informal basis the ARISE Intervention appears to be effective in engaging resistant patients and clients in treatment in these instances. In addition, where the primary problem is, for example, resisting regular testing of blood, urine, or blood pressure, attending regular doctor's appointments, or complying with prescribed medication, an Intervention Network coached by an Invitational Interventionist can bring about a remarkable change. When approached by a concerned other member of the support system about any of these problems, the Invitational Interventionist proceeds in much the same way as s/he would in dealing with a substance abuse issue. However, in each of the categories and sub-categories there are likely to be differences, ranging from subtle to blatant. It is useful to be aware of these differences and the need for specific training prior to offering one's services in any of these areas that may be less familiar to the Interventionist.

The authors hope that studies in the areas mentioned above will follow since they believe that the resources and resilience of families can be brought to bear on many of the problems that are currently costing significant and unnecessary mortality, morbidity, and expense to our population.

NOTE

1. National Institute on Drug Abuse–NIDA–RO1 DA09402.

REFERENCES

Azrin, N. H. (1976). Improvements in the community reinforcement approach to alcoholism. *Behavioral Research and Therapy, 14*, 339-348.

Barber, J. G., & Gilbertson, R. (1997). Unilateral interventions for women living with heavy drinkers. *Social Work, 42*(1), 69-77.

Festinger, D. W., Lamb, R. J., Kirby, K. C., & Marlowe, D. (1996). Accelerated intake: A method for reducing initial appointment no-shows for outpatient cocaine addiction treatment. *Journal of Applied Behavior Analysis, 29*, 357-389.

Frances, R. J., Miller, S. I., & Galanter, M. (1989). Psychosocial treatment of addictions. In A. Tasman, R. J. Hales, & A. Frances (Eds.), *Review of psychiatry* (Vol. 8; pp. 341-359). Washington, DC: American Psychiatric Press.

Galanter, M. (1993). *Network therapy for alcohol and drug abuse.* New York, NY: Basic Books.

Garrett, J., Landau-Stanton, J., Stanton, M. D., Stellato-Kabat, J., & Stellato-Kabat, D. (1997). ARISE: A method for engaging reluctant alcohol- and drug-dependent individuals in treatment. *Journal of Substance Abuse Treatment, 14*(3), 235-248.

Garrett, J., Landau, J., Stanton, M. D., Baciewicz, G., Brinkman-Sull, D., & Shea, R. (1998). The ARISE intervention: Using family links to overcome resistance to addiction treatment. *Journal of Substance Abuse Treatment, 15*(2), 333-343.

Garrett, J., Stanton, M. D., Landau, J., Baciewicz, G., Brinkman-Sull, D., & Shea, R. (1999). The "Concerned Other" call: Using family links to overcome resistance to addiction treatment. *Substance Use and Misuse, 34*(3), 363-382.

Garrett, J., & Landau, J. (2006). Family Motivation to Change: A major factor in engaging alcoholics in treatment. By invitation for special issue of *Alcoholism Treatment Quarterly, 24*(1/2).

Johnson, P. B., Richter, L., McLellan, A. T., & Kleber, H. D. (2002). Alcohol use patterns before and after September 11. *American Clinical Laboratory, 21*(7), 25-27.

Johnson, V. (1973). *I'll quit tomorrow.* New York: Harper & Row.

Kessler, R. C., McGonagle, K. A., Zhao, S., Nelson, C. B., Hughes, M., Eshleman, S., Wittchen, H-U., & Kendler, K. S. (1994). Lifetime and 12-month prevalence of DSM-III-R psychiatric disorders in the United States: Results from the National Comorbidity Survey. *Archives of General Psychiatry, 51*, 8-19.

Landau, J. (1979, July). *The black African family in transition.* Paper presented at the World Congress of the International Family Therapy Association, Tel Aviv, Israel.

Landau, J. (1981). Link therapy as a family therapy technique for transitional extended families. *Psychotherapeia*, October, 7(4).

Landau, J. (1982). Therapy with families in cultural transition. In M. McGoldrick, J. K. Pearce, & J. Giordano (Eds.), *Ethnicity and family therapy.* New York: Guilford Press.

Landau, J. (2004a, March). *Family motivation to change using invitational intervention in substance abuse treatment.* Paper presented at the 14th World Congress of the International Family Therapy Association on Families in Times of Global Crisis, Istanbul, Turkey.

Landau, J. (2004b, September). *Family motivation to change: Families and therapists as partners for addiction recovery.* Paper presented at the Annual Conference of The American Association for Marriage and Family Therapy, Atlanta, GA.

Landau, J. (2005). El modelo LINC: una estrategia colaborativa para la resiliencia comunitaria. *Sistemas Familiares, 20* (3); *www.e-libro.com.*

Landau, J., Garrett, J., Shea, R., Stanton, M. D., Baciewicz, G., & Brinkman-Sull, D. (2000). Strength in numbers: Using family links to overcome resistance to addiction treatment. *American Journal of Drug and Alcohol Abuse, 26*(3), 379-398.

Landau, J., & Garrett, J. (2006). *Invitational Intervention: A step by step guide for clinicians to help families engage resistant substance abusers in treatment.* BookSurge.com.

Landau, J., & Saul, J. (2004). Facilitating family & community resilience in response to major disaster. In F. Walsh & M. McGoldrick (Eds.). *Living beyond loss 2nd Ed.* New York: Norton.

Landau, J., & Stanton, M. D. (1990). *Alcoholism and addiction within the family: Intergenerational genesis, transmission, maintenance of symptoms, therapeutic implications.* Unpublished manuscript.

Landau, J., Stanton, M. D., Brinkman-Sull, D., Ikle, D., McCormick, D., Garrett, J., Baciewicz, G., Shea, R., & Wamboldt, F. (2004). Outcomes with *ARISE* approach to engaging reluctant drug- and alcohol-dependent individuals in treatment. *American Journal of Drug & Alcohol Abuse, 30*(4).

Landau-Stanton, J., & Clements, C. (1993). *AIDS, health and mental health: A primary sourcebook.* New York: Brunner/Mazel.

Loneck, B., Garrett, J., & Banks, S. (1996a). A comparison of the Johnson Intervention with four other methods of referral to outpatient treatment. *The American Journal of Drug and Alcohol Abuse, 22*(2), 233-246.

Loneck, B., Garrett, J., & Banks, S. (1996b). The Johnson Intervention and relapse during outpatient treatment. *The American Journal of Drug and Alcohol Abuse, 22*(3), 363-375.

Lystad, M. L. (Ed.) (1988). *Mental health response to mass emergencies: Theory and practice.* Brunner/Mazel: New York, NY.

Maher, W. (2006). *Verbal communication, February 22, 2006.*

McCrady, B. (2006). Family and other close relationships. In Wm. Miller & K. Carroll (Eds.). *Rethinking substance abuse.* Guilford Press. New York, NY.

Miller, W. R., & Myers, R. J. (1996). Unilateral family intervention for drug problems: Stage II trial (NIDA grant No. RO1 DA–08896-01). Albuquerque: University of New Mexico, Center for Alcoholism, Substance Abuse and Addictions.

Miller, W. R., Meyer, R. J., & Tonigan, J. S. (1999). Engaging the unmotivated in treatment for alcohol problems: A comparison of three intervention strategies. *Journal of Consulting and Clinical Psychology, 67,* 688-697.

Nathan, P. E. (1990). Prevention and early intervention of addictive disorders. In H. B. Milkman & L. I. Sederer (Eds.), *Treatment Choices for Alcoholism and Substance Abuse.* Lexington, MA: Lexington Books.

Perzel, J. F., & Lamon, S. (1979). *Enmeshment within families of polydrug abusers.* Paper presented at the National Drug Abuse Conference, New Orleans, August, 1979.

Raiter, W., & Toll, J. (2006). Presentation: "Systemic Intervention." Moment of Change Conference, Santa Monica, CA, February, 2006.

Rapaport, J. (1977). *Community Psychology: Values, research, and action.* Holt, Rinehart and Winston: New York, NY.

Seaburn, D., Landau-Stanton, J., & Horwitz, S. (1995). Core intervention techniques in family therapy process. In *Integrating Family Therapy: Handbook of family psychology and systems theory*; Mikesell, R.H., Lusterman, D.-D., McDaniel, S.H. (Eds.); American Psychological Association: Washington, DC, 1995; 5-26.

Sisson, R. W., & Azrin, N. H. (1986). Family-member involvement to initiate and promote treatment of problem drinkers. *Journal of Behavior Therapy and Experimental Psychiatry, 17,* 15-21.

Speck, R., & Attneave, C. (1973). *Family Networks.* New York: Pantheon Books.

Stanton, M. D., & Shadish, W. R. (1997). Outcome, attrition and family/couples treatment for drug abuse: A meta-analysis and review of the controlled, comparative studies. *Psychological Bulletin, 122*(2), 170-191.

Stasiewicz, P. R., & Stalker, R. (1999). A comparison of three "interventions" on pretreatment dropout rates in an outpatient substance abuse clinic. *Addictive Behaviors, 24,* 579-582.

Szapocznik, J., Perez-Vidal, A., Brickman, A. L., Foote, F. F., Santisteban, D., Hervis, O., & Kurtines, W. M. (1988). Engaging adolescent drug abusers and their families in treatment: A strategic structural systems approach. *Journal of Consulting and Clinical Psychology, 56*(4), 552-557.

Vaillant, G. E. (1995). *The natural history of alcoholism revisited.* Cambridge, MA: Harvard University Press.

doi:10.1300/J020v26n01_08

Working with Family Members
to Engage Treatment-Refusing Drinkers:
The CRAFT Program

Jane Ellen Smith, PhD
Robert J. Meyers, PhD
Julia L. Austin, MS

SUMMARY. Community Reinforcement and Family Training (CRAFT) is an empirically-supported program based on behavioral reinforcement that engages treatment-*refusing* alcohol-other drug abusers into treatment by working with their concerned family members. These concerned significant others (CSOs) are taught how to rearrange contingencies in the drinker's environment such that sober behavior is supported and drinking behavior is discouraged. CSOs receive behavioral skills training in order to acquire the tools to successfully influence the drinker to enter treatment, and to enhance their own happiness as well. This review describes the outgrowth of CRAFT from the original Community Reinforcement Approach (CRA) program, summarizes the research foundation, and presents

---

Jane Ellen Smith, Robert J. Meyers, and Julia L. Austin are all affiliated with the Psychology Department, and the Center on Alcoholism, Substance Abuse, and Addictions at the University of New Mexico, Albuquerque, NM.

Address correspondence to: Jane Ellen Smith, PhD, Department of Psychology, Logan 116, #1, University of New Mexico, Albuquerque, NM 87131-1161 (E-mail: janellen@unm.edu).

For further information, see website at http://casaa.unm.edu/craft.html.

[Haworth co-indexing entry note]: "Working with Family Members to Engage Treatment-Refusing Drinkers: The CRAFT Program." Smith, Jane Ellen, Robert J. Meyers, and Julia L. Austin. Co-published simultaneously in *Alcoholism Treatment Quarterly* (The Haworth Press) Vol. 26, No. 1/2, 2008, pp. 169-193; and: *Family Intervention in Substance Abuse: Current Best Practices* (ed: Oliver J. Morgan, and Cheryl H. Litzke) The Haworth Press, 2008, pp. 169-193. Single or multiple copies of this article are available for a fee from The Haworth Document Delivery Service [1-800-HAWORTH, 9:00 a.m. - 5:00 p.m. (EST). E-mail address: docdelivery@haworthpress.com].

the basic CRAFT procedures with illustrative examples. doi:10.1300/
J020v26n01_09 *[Article copies available for a fee from The Haworth Document
Delivery Service: 1-800-HAWORTH. E-mail address: <docdelivery@haworthpress.
com> Website: <http://www.HaworthPress.com> © 2008 by The Haworth Press.
All rights reserved.]*

KEYWORDS. Community reinforcement, treatment engagement, concerned significant others, contingency management

INTRODUCTION

When people in communities at large are asked: "Do you live with a relative or partner who has an alcohol problem but won't get help? Would *you* like help in dealing with this problem?" the response typically has been overwhelming. Perhaps this level of interest should not be surprising, given that individuals with an alcohol use disorder delay treatment for an average of 6-9 years after symptoms first begin (Wang et al., 2005). During those years, the drinker's loved ones are often exposed to various stressors, including financial difficulties, domestic violence, verbal aggression, poor family cohesion and inappropriate behavior from the using individual (Orford, Krishnan, & Velleman, 2003; Velleman et al., 1993). Understandably, the loved ones of individuals with a drinking problem are at an increased risk for depressive symptoms, lowered self-esteem, and physical problems (Brown, Kokin, Seraganian, & Shields, 1995). Although most drinkers seek to postpone treatment despite negative intra- and interpersonal consequences (Miller & Rollnick, 1991; Wang et al., 2005), their loved ones are usually anxious to initiate treatment in order to address the problems created by the drinking (Meyers, Smith, & Miller, 1998; Smith & Meyers, 2004). Community Reinforcement and Family Training (CRAFT) is a program with empirical backing that capitalizes on these family members as resources and extremely powerful agents of change.

CRAFT'S THEORETICAL FOUNDATION

Traditional Approaches

Until recently, these loved ones, or concerned significant others (CSOs), had only two available treatment options: the ubiquitous Al-Anon meeting (Al-Anon, 1984) or the Johnson Institute Intervention (Johnson, 1986). Al-Anon, which is based on 12-step philosophy, holds that CSOs are powerless over someone else's drinking. Al-Anon teaches CSOs to "lovingly detach" from the drinker and to cease any effort to control the drinker's behavior. In contrast, the Johnson Institute Intervention encourages CSOs to take an active role in attempting to get the drinker into treatment. CSOs are assisted in planning a surprise "intervention" in which a group of loved ones confronts the drinker about the negative impact of his or her behavior (Johnson, 1986). The Johnson Institute approach has become fashionable enough to inspire a reality television series on the Arts and Entertainment channel appropriately entitled, "Intervention." Despite being widespread, both Al-Anon and the Johnson Institute Intervention lack solid empirical support. In addition, both programs have characteristics which may run counter to the needs of many CSOs. Al-Anon is limited in that countless CSOs are unable or unwilling to "lovingly detach" from the drinker. Furthermore, CSOs often report difficulty implementing the Johnson Institute's confrontational approach (Barber & Gilbertson, 1997), which leads to small percentages of CSOs actually completing the intervention process (Liepman, Nirenberg, & Begin, 1989; Miller, Meyers, & Tonigan, 1999).

Unilateral Family Therapy

Unilateral family therapy (UFT) is a general descriptor for a type of treatment that works with family members *other than* the one with the identified problem. UFT is a relatively new alternative to the traditional approaches of Al-Anon and the Johnson Institute Intervention. The basic premise of UFT is that providing psychological treatment to CSOs can help facilitate non-drinking behaviors in the individual with a drinking problem (the identified patient; IP), as well as improve the CSOs' psychological functioning (Thomas & Santa, 1982). These approaches do not blame CSOs for their IP's drinking, but instead maintain that therapy can teach the CSOs strategies to help engage the IP into treatment. Different UFTs vary as to the specific skill sets they teach and the extent to which they emphasize confrontational techniques (see Smith & Meyers, 2004). Despite promising preliminary evidence as far as being able to engage substance abusers into treatment, most UFT approaches have yet to undergo rigorous examination. Further, research on UFTs is marred by case study designs (Garrett et al., 1998; Landau et al., 2000), the lack of adequate control groups (Landau et al., 2004) and non-random treatment assignment (Thomas & Ager, 1993; Thomas, Santa, Bronson, & Oyserman, 1987).

The UFT with the strongest empirical support is CRAFT. The CRAFT program is an extension of the Community Reinforcement Approach (CRA), which is a comprehensive, scientifically-supported behavioral intervention for the drinkers themselves (Azrin, 1976; Azrin, Sisson, Meyers, & Godley, 1982; Hunt & Azrin, 1973; Meyers & Smith, 1995; Smith, Meyers, & Delaney, 1998). Early CRA researchers noted that the family members of drinkers were invaluable collaborators in the treatment process. These family members spent a great deal of time with the drinking individual, were emotionally invested in helping the drinker get better, and had access to key reinforcers of both drinking and sober behavior (Meyers, Smith, & Lash, 2005). Thus, it followed naturally that a program should be developed in which CSOs were trained in behavioral principles to employ in their interactions with their IP at home.

Like CRA, CRAFT is based on operant theory, which holds that environmental contingencies play powerful roles in both the etiology of and recovery from substance abuse. CRAFT teaches CSOs to identify and rearrange their IP's contingencies, such that clean and sober behaviors become more rewarding than drinking behaviors. The objective of teaching CSOs these skill sets is to reduce the IP's substance abuse and to ultimately engage the IP in treatment. Note, however, that although CSOs are instrumental in creating positive changes, they are not held accountable for the IP's drinking or other negative behaviors. Importantly, in addition to addressing the IP's substance abuse, CRAFT provides CSOs with skills designed to improve their own psychological, physical, and social functioning.

CRAFT'S RESEARCH FOUNDATION

Earliest Alcohol Study

The first version of CRAFT, called CRT (Community Reinforcement Training), was tested in a small randomized trial with 12 female CSOs of male problem drinkers in rural Illinois (Sisson & Azrin, 1986). These CSOs were comprised of wives, sisters, and daughters of IPs who refused to seek treatment. The standard CRAFT protocol was used with the seven women assigned to CRT, whereas the five women assigned to standard treatment received individual counseling sessions based on the disease concept of alcoholism. The latter were also given referrals to

Al-Anon meetings, as well as an established procedure called Systematic Encouragement which had been proven to increase the likelihood of attendance at meetings (Sisson & Mallams, 1981). The main outcome of interest was IP treatment engagement.

A total of six of the seven CSOs (86%) who received CRT were able to get their IPs to seek alcohol treatment. In contrast, none of the IPs of the five CSOs in the comparison group began treatment. Interestingly, the CSOs of the six treatment-engaged individuals reported that the drinking actually had decreased significantly before the IP even started treatment; namely, during the time that just the CSO was in treatment. The drinking pattern appeared unchanged during this same time for the comparison group. The primary limitation of the study was the small sample size.

NIAAA-Funded Alcohol Trial

A large CRAFT study was not conducted until approximately 10 years later. This occurred in Albuquerque, NM, where 130 CSOs of treatment-refusing alcohol dependent individuals were recruited (Miller et al., 1999). The main *exclusion* criteria were that potential participants (CSOs): had contact with the IP on less than 40% of the days, were diagnosable substance abusers themselves, or had experienced serious domestic violence by the IP. CSOs were randomly assigned to CRAFT, Al-Anon Facilitation, or the Johnson Institute Intervention. Al-Anon Facilitation was modeled after the Project MATCH 12-step Facilitation Therapy (Nowinski, Baker, & Carroll, 1992), and consisted of an individual format for 12-step treatment that was aimed at promoting attendance at Al-Anon meetings. An added objective was IP treatment engagement. The Johnson Institute Intervention was as described earlier. Per its usual format, the Intervention entailed six 2-hour CSO sessions, whereas CSOs in the other two conditions were offered 12 one-hour sessions.

Overall, the CSOs included IP spouses (59%), parents (30%), girl-friends/boyfriends (8%), children (1.5%), and grandparents (1.5%). The majority of the CSOs (91%) were female. The CSO ethnic break-down was: white, non-Hispanic (53%), Hispanic (39%), Native American (6%), African American (1%), and "other" (1%). CSOs tended to be 47 years old, to have 14 years of education, and to be employed either full time (51%) or part time (17%). As far as attendance for the 12 hours of CSO treatment, there was no significant group difference between the completers among the CRAFT-trained CSOs (89%) and the Al-Anon Facilitation condition (95%). On the other hand, only 53% of the CSOs in the Intervention completed their allotted sessions. The main reason given for their premature termination was an unwillingness to go through with the family confrontation phase.

Treatment engagement was defined as an IP completing both the 4-hour intake and at least one therapy session. Significant differences in engagement were detected across conditions at the end of the 6-month window. CRAFT-trained CSOs engaged 64% of their IPs, the Johnson Institute Intervention engaged 30%, and the Al-Anon Facilitation condition engaged 13%. For the subset of drinkers who started treatment, the average number of sessions attended by their CSOs prior to treatment engagement was quite similar across conditions: CRAFT and the Johnson Institute Intervention were each 4.7 CSO sessions, and Al-Anon Facilitation was 5.7 sessions. The median number of sessions attended by the IPs once they began treatment was 10.5 out of a possible 12. Interestingly, the CRAFT-trained therapists were the least experienced, having between 0-3 years of experience with substance abusing clients.

As mentioned earlier, since CSOs understandably suffer from a variety of psychological problems (e.g., depression, relationship distress), one of the goals of CRAFT is to decrease CSO's own symptoms independent of the IP's outcome. In line with this objective, significant pre-post improvements were discovered across conditions for CSOs in terms of depression and anger, as well as for relationship issues characterized as family cohesion, conflict, and general relationship happiness. Importantly, these improvements occurred regardless of CSO treatment condition, and they were *not* limited to those CSOs who engaged their IPs in treatment (Miller et al., 1999).

CRAFT Illicit Drug Studies

A brief overview is presented of the three studies that were conducted with the CSOs of treatment-refusing IPs with illicit drug problems. Each study was funded by NIDA (National Institute on Drug Abuse). The program that was conducted in Philadelphia had a relatively small sample of CSOs (n = 32) who were randomly assigned to either individual CRAFT sessions or 12-step meetings (Kirby, Marlowe, Festinger, Garvey, & LaMonaca, 1999). Primarily the CSOs were women who were the IPs' spouses (56%) or parents (38%). The major ethnic breakdown of the CSOs was white (75%) and African American (22%). At the conclusion of the 10-week program, the CSOs who received CRAFT had engaged 64% of their treatment-refusing IPs into treatment, whereas the CSOs assigned to12-step meetings had engaged 17%. CSO functioning again improved regardless of treatment assignment.

An uncontrolled study with treatment-refusing drug abusers was conducted in Albuquerque in which all 62 CSOs received training in CRAFT (Meyers, Miller, Hill, & Tonigan, 1999). Overall, 74% of the IPs were engaged in treatment, and they completed an average of 7.6 of their 12 sessions. A large controlled trial was next conducted in Albuquerque with 90 CSOs of illicit drug users (Meyers, Miller, Smith, & Tonigan, 2002). CSOs were randomized to CRAFT, CRAFT + aftercare, or Al-Nar FT (Al-Anon–Nar-Anon Facilitation Therapy). Since the aftercare component did not enhance CRAFT treatment effects, it will not be discussed further. The engagement rate for the two CRAFT conditions combined was 67%, which was significantly better than for Al-Nar FT at 29%. IPs again attended 63% of their available sessions.

CRAFT PROCEDURES

Building Motivation and Rapport

When a CSO begins the CRAFT program, she or he tends to be motivated and highly invested in seeing the IP's drinking behavior change. This enthusiasm sometimes waivers a bit when, in the course of the CRAFT program description, CSOs discover that *they* are the ones who are going to have to do all of the hard work to influence this behavior change. It is important to acknowledge that although it is "unfair" for CSOs to have to make further sacrifices on behalf of the IP, the CSOs' big reward–namely, the IP getting into treatment–is dependent on the CSOs' continued commitment. You should refer to CSOs as crucial collaborators, both because they have a great deal of knowledge about their IP's drinking patterns, and they have considerable contact with the IP. Each of these factors is necessary in order to implement the CRAFT program, as it is grounded in learning principles. To illustrate this point, inform CSOs that they will learn how to appropriately offer positive reinforcement (rewards) for sober IP behavior, and to withdraw reinforcers for drinking.

There are other successful methods for increasing CSOs' resolve to work the CRAFT program while generally building rapport. For example, you should allow CSOs to express frustration, anger, and sadness as they review the numerous ways in which the IP's drinking has created problem after problem. You should also inquire about the CSOs' past attempts to halt the drinking, and then reinforce them for doing everything humanly possible to take care of their family. Once these issues have been discussed for a reasonable period of time, it is important to move the focus of the session to the future. The future is discussed in optimistic terms, primarily by describing the scientific backing for CRAFT. Specifically, CSOs are informed that: (1) CRAFT-trained individuals like themselves are successful at engaging treatment-refusing substance abusers into treatment nearly 7 out of 10 times, (2) treatment engagement occurs across a wide variety of CSO-IP relationships (e.g., spouses, parent and child, siblings), and for illicit drugs as well as for alcohol, and (3) CSOs tend to feel better emotionally (i.e., have less depression, anxiety, anger) after CRAFT *regardless* of whether their IP begins treatment (Smith & Meyers, 2004, p. 22). Tell CSOs that in addition to the obvious CRAFT goal of engaging the IP into treatment, there are actually two others: reducing the IP's drinking prior to treatment entry, and increasing CSOs' happiness independent of the IP's treatment status.

During the first session it is critical to highlight three points. First, confidentiality will be strictly upheld. It is fairly common for CSOs to refrain from telling their IPs that they are in therapy for several weeks, and consequently you must be particularly cautious about contacting CSOs. Furthermore, since domestic violence is sometimes a risk, CSO safety is a top priority (see "Domestic Violence Precautions"). Second, CSOs are *not* responsible for their IP's problematic drinking. Although CSOs' behavior at times may have inadvertently made it easier for their IP to drink, this is quite different from intentionally supporting the use of alcohol. This message is one that you will have to review periodically, such as when the CSOs' behavior is later explored in an effort to suggest alternative CSO responses to the IPs' drinking behavior. Third, progress toward treatment engagement unfolds over time after a series of behavioral changes occur on a consistent basis, and thus patience on the part of the CSO is imperative.

CRAFT Functional Analysis

A core assumption of CRAFT is that CSOs can learn to modify their behavior in ways that will help IPs reduce their drinking. In order to provide specific and well-informed suggestions to CSOs regarding changing their interactions with their IP, you must ask CSOs to identify the typical context for the IP's drinking behavior by conducting a CRAFT Functional Analysis (see Appendix A for the functional analysis chart used by CRAFT clinicians). This functional analysis is unique, inasmuch as it describes the purpose (i.e., the function) of the drinker's behavior . . . but it does so from the perspective of someone other than the drinker. Once the factors that appear to be maintaining the IP's drinking behavior are uncovered, the foundation is in place to develop a plan of action for the CSO to intervene.

As part of the functional analysis, ask CSOs to describe the IP's normal use pattern, including the typical external cues (places, people, or times) and internal cues (thoughts and feelings) that are associated with their IP's drinking behavior. You should explain that cues (triggers) are not only the factors that immediately precede the drinking behavior, but also the more distal factors that may have set the stage for use. Labeling these typical triggers as high risk situations is a significant step toward eventually developing a plan of action for the CSO. For instance, if it becomes apparent that an IP's main internal trigger to drink is boredom, then the CSO can generate strategies for helping the IP develop and choose alternative, healthy activities to replace drinking as a response to boredom.

By examining the short-term positive consequences of drinking, the functional analysis highlights the ways in which the IP's drinking behavior is positively or negatively reinforcing. The objective is to identify substitute behaviors that may serve similar functions as alcohol use, and then to determine whether the CSO can play a role in facilitating the choice of these behaviors. For example, assume the functional analysis reveals that the IP often appears more relaxed after drinking alcohol. You could explore with the CSO several alcohol-free methods which have resulted in stress reduction for the IP in the past, and see whether the CSO can play a role in re-introducing and supporting any of these methods. The final segment of the functional analysis consists of reviewing the negative long-term effects of the IP's alcohol use (e.g., family conflict, financial distress, health problems). In addition to outlining IP reinforcers to target that have been "damaged" or lost, a review of these negative consequences, perhaps surprisingly, frequently reinvigorates a discouraged CSO.

Domestic Violence Precautions

There is ample evidence to suggest that alcohol abuse is associated with aggressive behaviors (Collins, 1981; Greenfeld, 1998), including domestic violence (Fals-Stewart, 2003; Fals-Stewart & Kennedy, 2005; Gondolf & Foster, 1991; O'Farrell & Murphy, 1995; Stith, Crossman, & Bischof, 1991). Since CRAFT entails having CSOs make environmental changes which IPs may find uncomfortable, it is especially important to assess domestic violence risk. During the initial session, violence risk should be assessed by an instrument such as the Conflict Tactics Scale (Straus, 1979), or by a standard interview.

If a history of aggressive behavior is found, it is useful to further explore the patterns of this behavior with a modified functional analysis. One goal of a functional analysis for an IP's physically aggressive behavior is to help the CSO identify the typical antecedents (e.g., the IP acting distant, screaming, rubbing hands together). You would help the CSO initiate new, safer responses to these antecedents, such as ending the conversation, or even leaving home for a few hours. Role-plays are utilized so that the CSO can practice these new responses, and barriers to engaging in these responses can be addressed. In cases where the assessment reveals a more serious history of domestic violence, it is vital to minimize any immediate risk to the CSO. Occasionally you might decide that it is imprudent to proceed with CRAFT given the volatile nature of the CSO-IP relationship. Alternatively, it may be preferable to help the CSO design a safety plan, such as knowing how to obtain a restraining order. Throughout this process it is crucial to determine CSOs' level of social support, since they may need to garner assistance from their support system during future crises (Smith & Meyers, 2004, pp. 99-104).

Positive Communication Skills

One key difference between CRAFT and both Al-Anon and the Johnson Institute Intervention is that CRAFT emphasizes the importance of positive communication skills. The typical CSOs who seek out CRAFT are individuals who wish to maintain a relationship with their IP, thereby making it vital to help these CSOs learn to communicate in a positive manner. By the time they begin therapy, many CSOs have faced years of embarrassing behavior and broken promises. Understandably, frustration with their IP's behavior is often expressed at home in an irritated or angry manner. In contrast, some CSOs and IPs do not speak to each other at all anymore. Given that CRAFT asks CSOs to make environmental changes that may initially upset the IP, it is especially important that CSOs are able to express themselves in an assertive, non-hostile manner.

Much like behavioral couples therapy (Epstein & McCrady, 1998; O'Farrell & Fals-Stewart, 2003), CRAFT teaches basic rules for positive communication. CSOs are taught to: (1) be brief, (2) be positive, (3) be specific and clear, (4) label their feelings, (5) offer an understanding statement, (6) accept partial responsibility [for the *non*-drinking problem being addressed], and (7) offer to help. These behaviors are modeled for CSOs, and strengthened through the use of role-plays and positive reinforcement.

Positive Reinforcement of Non-Drinking Behaviors

Upon introducing the idea of positive reinforcement, it is common for CSOs to ask with some trepidation, "But isn't that enabling?" It is useful to contrast the critical difference between the two terms. "Enabling" represents a CSO behavior that increases IP drinking, whereas CRAFT's positive reinforcement, by definition, involves the CSO rewarding a *non*-drinking behavior or activity. Once this distinction is made, you should explain that a rewarded behavior tends to increase. And since CSOs would be rewarding *non*-drinking behaviors, these should not only increase, but they could then compete with drinking behaviors for time in the IP's schedule.

The next step involves presenting the guidelines for identifying suitable reinforcers. In brief, the reinforcers should be enjoyable for the IP, free or otherwise affordable, available to deliver as needed, and comfortable for the CSO to deliver (see Smith & Meyers, 2004, p. 138). Assume that a CSO lives with her sister: a young woman who opens up a new bottle of wine every day after work (IP). In settling on a positive reinforcer, the CSO states that she would like to make her sister a special meal every night that the IP comes home and does not drink. All suggestions for reinforcers, including this very generous one, must be reviewed for suitability. In this case the CSO would likely have insufficient time, money, and energy for such an undertaking. A more reasonable positive reinforcer might be for the CSO to spend pleasant time with the IP on the evenings that she does not drink. This would be narrowed down to several previously shared recreational activities such as watching TV, playing cards, looking through old photo albums, or calling mutual friends. To check for adherence to the guidelines you still would need to determine if spending time together engaged in these activities was something that the IP (and CSO) enjoyed, and whether the CSO's schedule permitted this level of involvement.

Since it is critical for the reinforcer to be given in response to sober behavior, check to be certain that CSOs are capable of detecting when their IP has *not* been drinking (see Smith & Meyers, 2004, pp. 147-8). Furthermore, prepare CSOs to inform their IP as to why they are providing a reinforcer at that particular time. Some CSOs intentionally delay having this conversation, and instead experiment with the behavior changes alone first. Nevertheless, it is necessary for CSOs to be ready for the conversation, since IPs sometimes ask why the CSO has started behaving differently around the house. The CSO from the scenario above would have practiced positive communication skills in order to say something to the effect of, "You're right; I have been acting differently lately. I'm trying to show you how much I *love* spending time with you when you're sober (feelings labeled; stated in a positive way). In fact, I'd be happy to do just about anything to help you stay cheerful like you are tonight without alcohol" (an offer to help).

The Use of Negative Consequences for Drinking Behaviors

The introduction of reinforcers for sober behavior has a natural complement: removing rewards for drinking. In fact, it frequently is impossible to do the former correctly without also implementing the latter. To illustrate: the CSO (sister) planned to engage in a pleasant activity with her sister when the IP did not drink. The unstated assumption is that the CSO would *not* engage in a pleasant activity with the sister if she drank. In essence, the CSO would be withdrawing a reinforcer (spending pleasant time with the sister) that had been in operation. However, this contingency needs to be clearly outlined, since most CSOs readily agree to the notion of positive reinforcement (once it is disentangled from enabling), but many initially balk at the idea of removing rewards. CSOs tend to voice less concern if the reward they are expected to withdraw on drinking occasions is a novel one that has been introduced specifically to reward sober behavior. Additionally, CSOs commonly report feeling more comfortable with the thought of withdrawing a reward if they can "warn" the IP in advance. This is perfectly acceptable, but it does require role-plays of the proposed communication with the IP. Regardless, it is worthwhile to remind CSOs that each CRAFT procedure is designed to move them toward their objective of getting their IP to enter treatment; which is the *CSOs'* reward.

A second method for identifying important occasions for withdrawing rewards entails watching for ways in which CSOs are reinforcing drinking behaviors unintentionally on an ongoing basis. This information is often revealed in the CRAFT Functional Analysis when the positive consequences of drinking are outlined. If it is not listed on the functional analysis and this CSO behavior has not otherwise become apparent, simply ask CSOs directly about their response to the IP's drinking. As an example of an appropriate reward to withdraw, imagine that each time a husband (IP) experiences a morning hangover his wife (CSO) makes him a special breakfast to help him feel better. You would gently explore this CSO behavior in an effort to help her realize that although she is not responsible for the husband's drinking, she could proactively take steps that would make it slightly more difficult for him to choose to drink the next time. Using the proper wording for this CRAFT procedure is paramount, because CSOs already frequently believe that if only they were not "inadequate" in some way, their IP would stop drinking. Therefore it is necessary to proceed carefully with this difficult and yet extremely important discussion. Reassurances about the CSOs' dedication to the family's well-being are especially beneficial here.

When it is time to develop a precise strategy to avoid rewarding the drinking-related behavior in the future, you can use a structured 8-step problem-solving procedure to generate a plan (see Smith & Meyers, 2004, pp. 187-198 for details). The current version (see Appendix B for the Problem Solving Worksheet used by CRAFT clinicians) is a modification of a procedure developed years ago by D'Zurilla and Goldfried (1971). Briefly, the problem above would be defined (step 1) as the wife needing an alternative response to making her husband a special breakfast on his hangover mornings; a response that would not be interpreted by the husband as reinforcing his drinking in any manner. The brainstorming segment (step 2) entails generating a variety of possible solutions to the problem (e.g., making a "non-special" breakfast, making no breakfast at all, leaving a note and going to mom's that morning, telling husband about therapy and inviting him to attend). Constructing a sizable list requires both the CSO's and your own input. The CSO next eliminates any of the suggestions that she cannot imagine herself attempting in the upcoming week, regardless of the reason (step 3). She settles on one of the remaining solutions (making a "non-special" breakfast), and describes exactly how she will carry it out (step 4).

Oftentimes potential obstacles to enacting the solution become apparent during the 4th step, but in the event that they do not, you should ask explicitly about any barriers (step 5). For instance, assume the CSO anticipates that her husband will pressure her to make his special breakfast anyway, and she will not know what to tell him. If the CSO is ready to explain her behavior to him, you would do several role-plays in which you practice a positive communication about the topic. One such conversation might be, "Honey, I enjoy making special treats for you, but it doesn't feel right anymore to do it on the mornings after you've been drinking. Instead I'd like to make my special breakfasts on the weekend mornings after you *haven't* been drinking. I hope you understand that I am doing this because I love you." Note that this solution changes the contingencies so that not only is the reward withdrawn when the IP is drinking, but his sober behavior is now rewarded. If each potential obstacle cannot be addressed, a different solution should be selected (step 6). Before ending the exercise the CSO should fully describe the plan for the new behavior (step 7). The final step of the problem-solving procedure is for you to check on the outcome in the next session, and to work with the CSO to make any required modifications to the plan (step 8).

CRAFT also teaches CSOs to allow the natural consequences of drinking behavior to occur–to a reasonable degree. Many CSOs intervene in an attempt to "fix" a problem created by the drinking behavior, thereby unwittingly protecting their IP from the natural negative consequences of drinking. For example, CSOs make excuses for missed family events, or clean up messes created by intoxicated IPs. Importantly, CSOs who exhibit these behaviors have the best intentions; they simply do not know how to successfully use the "power" they have in their relationship with the IP. In discussing this topic, emphasize again that nobody questions the sincerity of their commitment to seeing the IP improve, and that their pattern of intervening to prevent a negative consequence is actually a natural, loving response. However, since intervening in this manner does not *change* a problem behavior, you are going to help them develop a different type of loving response; one that will curb the IP's drinking. If CSOs have trouble isolating instances in which they are failing to allow the natural negative consequences of drinking to occur, you could revisit the functional analysis section on positive consequences of drinking. In reality, the natural consequences procedure is usually introduced when a blatant example of a CSO blocking the negative consequences surfaces.

There is one significant caveat to consider when teaching procedures that involve the use of negative consequences. It is imperative that you explore in advance any possible negative repercussions that CSOs might suffer once they withdraw reinforcement or allow for natural negative consequences of their IP's drinking. Since IPs may be angered by their CSO's new behavior, you must watch for warning signs of domestic violence, and review established safety procedures if indicated (see "Domestic Violence Precautions"). In addition to concerns about the CSOs' physical safety, you must also consider the gravity of the consequences in general for the CSO and the rest of the family. If it is obvious that an IP is going to lose a job as a result of the CSO no longer calling in excuses for him when he has a hangover, then this consequence with its wide-reaching financial effects on the entire family is probably best left untouched. Similarly, if IPs are certain to drive home drunk if their CSOs do not pick them up, then the CSOs would *not* be encouraged to allow the natural consequence. In cases such as these, an alternative CRAFT procedure would be utilized.

Multi-Faceted Enrichment of CSOs' Own Lives

As noted from the outset, increasing the quality of the CSO's life, re-gardless of what happens to the IP, is one of the main goals of CRAFT. After all, the CSO is your client, and so your client's well-being overall is of utmost concern. And although most CSOs feel happier once their IP reduces drinking and/or enters treatment, there is no absolute guaran-tee that these will occur. Furthermore, when encouraged to take a good look at specific aspects of their own lives, many CSOs decide that there are areas in which they would like to see "movement." A common first focus is the CSOs' self-imposed isolation that is an outgrowth of the complications associated with living with a heavy drinker. The tools for facilitating CSO changes already have been taught in some instances, and the remaining ones are borrowed from the Community Reinforce-ment Approach (CRA; Hunt & Azrin, 1973; Meyers & Smith, 1995).

Having a CSO complete a Happiness Scale is an excellent starting point (see Smith & Meyers, 2004, p. 223). This one-page clinical instru-ment asks clients to indicate on a scale from 1 (completely unhappy) to 10 (completely happy) how happy they are currently with their lives in various categories (see Appendix C). Some of the 10 categories include: social life, job/education, and personal habits. Your objective is to pin-point areas of CSOs' lives where they might want to make some changes in order to be happier. Initially it is prudent to steer clear of the most problematic areas (e.g., marriage) to increase the likelihood that CSOs will experience some progress quickly. Once a category has been selected, help set a goal toward achieving greater life satisfaction.

The CRA Goals of Counseling form (see Smith & Meyers, 2004, pp. 224-5) is designed to mirror the same life categories as the Happi-ness Scale. Nevertheless, any standard treatment plan can serve the same function; the structure of the goals themselves is the more impor-tant issue. The basic guidelines for goal-setting should sound familiar to any cognitive-behavioral therapist. In sum, the goals and the strategies for obtaining them should be: brief (uncomplicated), positive (what *will* be done; not what *won't* be done anymore), specific (measurable), reasonable, under the CSO's control, and based on skills the CSO possesses or is acquiring in treatment.

Assume a father (CSO) has sought CRAFT training to deal with a treatment-refusing alcohol-dependent teenage son (IP). Imagine that in the course of the previous year the CSO gradually eliminated all of his own social activities, and instead stays home and worries about his son. In examining the father's Happiness Scale you notice that he rated Social Life a "5." When you inquire as to what would raise that rating to a "6" or "7," the CSO states that he misses his fishing trips with his buddies on the weekend. If he agrees to work on this category, you would help him set a short-term goal and an initial strategy for achieving it. Assume he states his goal as: "to go fishing with my two buddies again." You would first reinforce his efforts to establish a goal, and note that it was brief, positive, and based on skills he possesses. Next you would help him shape the goal to conform to the remaining guidelines. This would entail making it more specific (e.g., "every Saturday morning"), and yet reasonable (e.g., "every other Saturday morning"). As far as it being under the CSO's control, assume the only obstacle is his fear that his son might need him in the event of an alcohol-related emergency. You could introduce problem-solving to address this issue. If the selected solution is for the CSO to buy a cell phone, this would be designated as part of the strategy for accomplishing the fishing trip goal. An additional step might include the CSO contacting his friends and explaining why he has been turning down their invitations. You would assess via role-play whether communication training was needed in order to successfully carry out this step. As always, progress toward the goal would be monitored so that obstacles could be addressed along the way.

The Invitation to Enter Treatment

Preparing CSOs to extend the invitation for their IP to enter treatment begins with CSOs' earliest involvement in CRAFT. The expectation is that the foundation will be well in place at the time the request is made. Building this foundation obviously includes teaching CSOs the positive communication skills to present the treatment request. However, each of the CRAFT procedures plays a role in the preparation, because IPs seem to be more likely to accept an invitation to begin treatment if they have already reduced their drinking somewhat by the time the request is made. Thus, the CSOs' new skills for appropriately giving and withdrawing positive reinforcement serve an essential function, as does learning problem-solving skills to address any associated issues. Consequently, it is necessary to slow down the overly zealous CSOs so that they do not simply rush home and extend yet another [unsuccessful] treatment request. Given that the average length of time it takes for IPs to enter treatment is less than five CSO sessions (Meyers et al., 1999, 2002; Miller et al., 1999), the majority of CSOs do not have long to wait.

There is no one right occasion for inviting an IP to enter treatment, but certain times are definitely better than others. CSOs are asked to identify the most promising times and places for approaching their IP in general, as these are frequently reasonable occasions for the treatment request. Importantly, the occasion should be a time when the IP is sober. Universal windows of opportunity should be discussed as well. These are noteworthy IP behaviors that seem to characterize a more open IP attitude. Samples of these are: (1) the IP behaving remorseful for having caused an alcohol-related crisis (e.g., DWI, assault; Bombardier, Ehde, & Kilmer, 1997; Longabaugh et al., 1995), (2) the IP asking why the CSO's behavior has changed, usually in response to the CSO rewarding sober behavior suddenly, and (3) the IP asking what happens in the CSO's sessions (when the IP knows about the CSO's therapy).

In terms of *how* to invite IPs to begin treatment, based on the CRAFT studies there appear to be motivational "hooks" that CSOs can use to make the prospect of therapy more appealing (Miller, Ogle, Anderson, Meyers, & Miller, 1999). A selection of these include informing IPs that: (1) they can have their own therapist; a therapist other than their CSO's therapist, (2) they do not have to focus exclusively on alcohol in therapy, but can work on a variety of problems (e.g., finding a new job, depression), (3) they will have major input into the treatment process and goals, and (4) they can "sample" treatment by attending a session or two, and if they do not care for it they can discontinue. One representative request by a woman (CSO) to have her partner (IP) enter treatment is: "I know that work is really stressful for you (positive communication skills: understanding statement) and you drink to relax after a rough day, but I bet there's a healthier way to relax that could also be fun. My therapist says you could see your own counselor (motivational hook # 1 above); somebody who would help you figure out ways to relax and have fun without drinking, and who'd also see about reducing the stress of your job (motivational hook # 2 above). Would you be willing to try it just once (motivational hook # 4 above) . . . for us?"

Of course, in order to make promises regarding the content of an IP's treatment, you must be confident that a treatment program is available that can deliver on the promises. Cognitive behavioral programs for substance abusers in general would be suitable, and CRA in particular

(Azrin et al., 1982; Meyers & Smith, 1995). Consistent with the CRAFT rapid intake model, being available also implies that the program for the IP should be ready to accept new clients within 48 hours of IPs stating that they want to begin treatment. Therapists within agencies often make arrangements to pick up IP cases for each other without delay.

In the process of rehearsing the treatment invitation, you should discuss the realistic possibility that despite the most polished conversation, the IP could still refuse. Alternatively, the IP may agree to enter treatment, but then drop out prematurely. CSOs need to be prepared to face these outcomes, and to have a plan for following up in the aftermath. Additionally, CSOs should be cognizant of the importance of their continued commitment to deliver various CRAFT procedures even when the IP is in treatment, as these crucial changes at home will support the IP's progress.

CONCLUDING RECOMMENDATIONS

For those practitioners who decide that they are interested in implementing CRAFT, a few suggestions are offered:

- Most therapists would benefit from obtaining comprehensive instructions regarding how to conduct CRAFT, and thus you might consider getting a copy of the therapists' manual: *Motivating Substance Abusers to Enter Treatment: Working with Family Members* (Smith & Meyers, 2004). Furthermore, it is highly recommended that you also get the companion book for clients (CSOs): *Get Your Loved One Sober: No More Nagging, Pleading, and Threatening* (Meyers & Wolfe, 2004).
- Keep in mind that CRAFT's style is motivational rather than confrontational. Specifically, it relies on the CSO's skillful introduction of rewards for sober IP behavior. At the same time, CSOs also learn to withdraw rewards in response to IP drinking. Positive communication skills are viewed as integral to the proper implementation of CRAFT, and thus are stressed throughout the CSO's treatment.
- Novice CRAFT therapists would probably find it worthwhile to have contact with other CRAFT-trained therapists. In part, this is because one must be unusually creative at times in order to help CSOs design a plan for influencing behavior change in a treatment resistant loved one. Thus, suggestions from other CRAFT therapists

are always appreciated. Additionally, regular contact with CRAFT therapists can serve as a motivator so that you do not become complacent in your efforts to assist clients in engaging their loved ones into treatment.

- Remember the basics about CRAFT. This program has proven to be successful at engaging treatment-*refusing* substance abusers into treatment in 64%-86% of the cases. Furthermore, the CSOs in these studies represent a wide variety of ethnic backgrounds, and their relationship with the IP has included being the IP's parent, spouse, adult child, romantic partner, and friend. Treatment engagement usually occurs quickly, in less than five CSO sessions. For CSOs it tends to be a "win/win" situation, given that their psychosocial functioning typically improves regardless of whether their IP ever becomes engaged in treatment.

REFERENCES

Al-Anon Family Groups. (1984). *Al-Anon faces alcoholism.* New York: Author.

Azrin, N. (1976). Improvements in the community reinforcement approach to alcoholism. *Behaviour Research and Therapy, 14,* 339-348.

Azrin, N., Sisson, R. W., Meyers, R. J., & Godley, M. (1982). Alcoholism treatment by disulfiram and community reinforcement therapy. *Journal of Behaviour Therapy and Experimental Psychiatry, 13,* 105-112.

Barber, J. G., & Gilbertson, R. (1997). Unilateral interventions for women living with heavy drinkers. *Social Work, 42,* 69-78.

Bombardier, C. H., Ehde, D., & Kilmer, J. (1997). Readiness to change alcohol drinking habits after traumatic brain injury. *Archives of Physical Medicine and Rehabilitation, 78,* 592-596.

Brown, T. G., Kokin, M., Seraganian, P., & Shields, N. (1995). Models of helping and coping. *American Psychologist, 37,* 368-384.

Collins, J. J. Jr. (1981). Alcohol use and criminal behavior: An empirical, theoretical, and methodological overview. In J. J. Collins Jr. (Ed.), *Drinking and crime: Perspectives on the relationships between alcohol consumption and criminal behavior.* New York: Guilford Press.

D'Zurilla, T. J., & Goldfried, M. R. (1971). Problem solving and behavior modification. *Journal of Abnormal Psychology, 78,* 107-126.

Epstein, E. E., & McCrady, B. S. (1998). Behavioral couples treatment of alcohol and drug use disorders: Current status and innovations. *Clinical Psychology Review, 18,* 689-711.

Fals-Stewart, W. (2003). The occurrence of partner physical aggression on days of alcohol consumption: A longitudinal diary study. *Journal of Consulting and Clinical Psychology, 71,* 41-52.

Fals-Stewart, W., & Kennedy, C. (2005). Addressing intimate partner violence in substance-abuse treatment. *Journal of Substance Abuse Treatment, 29,* 5-17.
Garrett, J., Landau, J., Shea, R., Stanton, M. D., Baciewicz, G., & Brinkman-Sull, D.
(1998). The ARISE intervention: Using family and network links to engage addicted persons in treatment. *Journal of Substance Abuse Treatment, 15,* 333-343.
Gondolf, E. W., & Foster, R. A. (1991). Wife assault among VA alcohol rehabilitation
patients. *Hospital and Community Psychiatry, 42,* 74-79.
Greenfeld, L. A. (1998). *Alcohol and crime: An analysis of national data on the preva-
lence of alcohol involvement in crime.* Report prepared for Assistant Attorney Gen-
eral's National Symposium on Alcohol Abuse and Crime. Washington, DC: U.S.
Department of Justice.
Hunt, G. M., & Azrin, N. H. (1973). A community reinforcement approach to alcohol-
ism. *Behaviour Research and Therapy, 11,* 91-104.
Johnson, V. E. (1986). *Intervention: How to help those who don't want help.* Minneapolis:
Johnson Institute.
Kirby, K. C., Marlowe, D. B., Festinger, D. S., Garvey, K. A., & LaMonaca, V. (1999).
Community reinforcement training for family and significant others of drug abus-
ers: A unilateral intervention to increase treatment entry of drug users. *Drug and Al-
cohol Dependence, 56,* 85-96.
Landau, J., Garrett, J., Shea, R. R., Stanton, M. D., Baciewicz, G., & Brinkman-Sull, D.
(2000). Strength in numbers: Using family links to overcome resistance to addiction
treatment. *American Journal of Drug and Alcohol Abuse, 26,* 379-398.
Landau, J., Stanton, M. D., Brinkman-Sull, D., Ikle, D., McCormick, D., Garrett, J.,
Baciewicz, G., Shea, R., Browning, A., & Wamboldt, F. (2004). Outcomes with the
ARISE approach to engaging reluctant drug- and alcohol-dependent individuals in
treatment. *American Journal of Drug & Alcohol Abuse, 30,* 711-748.
Liepman, M. R., Nirenberg, T. D., & Begin, A. M. (1989). Evaluation of a program designed to help family and significant others to motivate resistant alcoholics into re-
covery. *American Journal of Drug and Alcohol Abuse, 15,* 209-221.
Longabaugh, R., Minugh, A., Nirenberg, T., Clifford, P., Becker, B., & Woolard, R.
(1995). Injury as a motivator to reduce drinking. *Academy of Emergency Medicine,
2,* 817-825.
Meyers, R. J., Miller, W. R., Hill, D. E., & Tonigan, J. S. (1999). Community reinforcement and family training (CRAFT): Engaging unmotivated drug users in treatment.
Journal of Substance Abuse, 10, 1-18.
Meyers, R. J., Miller, W. R., Smith, J. E., & Tonigan, J. S. (2002). A randomized trial of
two methods for engaging treatment-refusing drug users through concerned significant others. *Journal of Consulting and Clinical Psychology, 70,* 1182-1185.
Meyers, R. J., & Smith, J. E. (1995). *Clinical guide to alcohol treatment: The community reinforcement approach.* New York: Guilford Press.
Meyers, R. J., Smith, J. E., & Lash, D. N. (2005). A program for engaging treatment-refusing substance abusers into treatment: CRAFT. *International Journal of Behavioral and Consultation Therapy, 1,* 90-100.
Meyers, R. J., Smith, J. E, & Miller, E. J. (1998). Working through the concerned
significant other: Community reinforcement and family training. In W. R. Miller

& N. Heather (Eds.), *Treating addictive behaviors: Processes of change.* New York: Plenum Press.

Meyers, R. J., & Wolfe, B. L. (2004). *Get your loved one sober: Alternatives to nagging, pleading, and threatening.* Center City, MN: Hazelden.

Miller, E., Ogle, R., Anderson, R., Meyers, R., & Miller, W. (1999, November). *Barriers to treatment and reasons for seeking treatment.* Poster presented at the meeting of the Association for Advancement of Behavior Therapy, Toronto, Canada.

Miller, W. R., Meyers, R. J., & Tonigan, J. S. (1999). Engaging the unmotivated in treatment for alcohol problems: A comparison of three strategies for intervention through family members. *Journal of Consulting and Clinical Psychology, 67,* 688-697.

Miller, W. R., & Rollnick, S. (1991). *Motivational interviewing: Preparing people to change addictive behavior.* New York: Guilford Press.

Nowinski, J., Baker, S., & Carroll, K. (1992). *12-step facilitation therapist manual: A clinical research guide for therapists treating individuals with alcohol abuse and dependence.* (Project MATCH Monograph Series, Vol. 1). Rockville, MD: National Institute on Alcohol Abuse and Alcoholism.

O'Farrell, T. J., & Murphy, C. M. (1995). Marital violence before and after alcoholism treatment. *Journal of Consulting and Clinical Psychology, 63,* 256-262.

O'Farrell, T. J., & Fals-Stewart, W. (2003). Marital and family therapy. In R. K. Hester and W. R. Miller (Eds.), *Handbook of alcoholism treatment approaches: Effective alternatives.* (3rd ed.). Boston: Allyn and Bacon.

Orford, J., Krishnan, M., & Velleman, R. (2003) Young adult offspring of parents with drinking problems: A study of childhood family cohesion using simple family diagrams. *Journal of Substance Use, 8,* 139-149.

Sisson, R. W., & Azrin, N. H. (1986). Family-member involvement to initiate and promote treatment of problem drinkers. *Behavior Therapy and Experimental Psychiatry, 17,* 15-21.

Sisson, R. W., & Mallams, J. H. (1981). The use of systematic encouragement and community access procedures to increase attendance at Alcoholics Anonymous and Al-Anon meetings. *American Journal of Drug and Alcohol Abuse, 8,* 371-376.

Smith, J. E., & Meyers, R. J. (2004). *Motivating substance abusers to enter treatment: Working with family members.* New York: Guilford.

Smith, J. E., Meyers, R. J., & Delaney, H. D. (1998). The community reinforcement approach with homeless alcohol-dependent individuals. *Journal of Consulting and Clinical Psychology, 66,* 541-548.

Stith, S. M., Crossman, R. K., & Bischof, G. P. (1991). Alcoholism and marital violence: A comparative study of men in alcohol treatment programs and batterer treatment programs. *Alcoholism Treatment Quarterly, 8,* 3-20.

Straus, M. A. (1979). Measuring intrafamily conflict and violence: The Conflict Tactics Scales. *Journal of Marriage and the Family, 41,* 75-86.

Thomas, E. J., & Ager, R. D. (1993). Unilateral family therapy with spouses of uncooperative alcohol abusers. In T.J. O'Farrell (Ed.), *Treating alcohol problems: Marital and family interventions.* New York: Guilford Press.

Thomas, E. J., & Santa, C. A. (1982). Unilateral family therapy for alcohol abuse: A working conception. *American Journal of Family Therapy, 10,* 49-58.

Thomas, E. J ., Santa, C., Bronson, D., & Oyserman, D. (1987). Unilateral family therapy with spouses of alcoholics. *Journal of Social Service Research, 10,* 145-163.

Velleman, R., Bennett, G., Miller, T., Orford, J., Rigby, K., & Tod, A. (1993). The families of problem drug users: A study of 50 close relatives. *Addiction, 88,* 1281-1289.

Wang, P. S., Berglund, P., Olfson, M. Pincus, H. A., Wells, K. B., & Kessler, R. C. (2005). Failure and delay in initial treatment contact after first onset of mental disorders in the national comorbidity survey replication. *Archives of General Psychiatry, 62,* 603-613.

doi:10.1300/J020v26n01_09

APPENDIX A

CRAFT FUNCTIONAL ANALYSIS FOR A LOVED ONE'S DRINKING/USING BEHAVIOR

External Triggers	Internal Triggers	Drinking/Using Behavior	Short-Term Positive Consequences	Long-Term Negative Consequences
1. Who is your loved one usually with when drinking/using?	1. Do you have any idea what your loved one is thinking about right before drinking/using?	1. What does your loved one usually drink/use?	1. What do you think your loved one likes about drinking/using with (who)?	1. What do you think are the negative results of your loved one drinking/using in each of one drinking/using in each of these areas (* the ones he/she would agree with):
				a) Interpersonal:
			2. What do you think he/she likes about drinking/using (where)?	b) Physical:
2. Where does he/she usually drink/use?	2. Do you have any idea what he/she is usually feeling right before drinking/using?	2. How much does he/she usually drink/use?	3. What do you think he/she likes about drinking/using (when)?	c) Emotional:
				d) Legal:
			4. Do you have any idea what pleasant thoughts he/she has while drinking/using?	e) Job:
3. When does he/she usually drink/use?		3. Over how long a period of time does he/she usually drink/use?	5. Do you have any idea what pleasant feelings he/she has while drinking/using?	f) Financial:
				g) Other:

Source: Motivating Substance Abusers to Enter Treatment: Working with Family Members (pp. 74-75) by J. E. Smith & R. J. Meyers, 2004, New York: Guilford Press. [Copyright 2004 by Guilford Press. Adapted by permission.]

APPENDIX B

Problem Solving Worksheet

1. <u>Define the problem</u>. [Just one…..and keep it real specific. Write it out below.]

2. <u>Brainstorm possible solutions</u>. [The more the better! Let yourself go here! List below.]

3. <u>Eliminate unwanted suggestions</u>. [Cross out any that don't seem practical/helpful]
4. <u>Select one potential solution</u>. [Which one looks really good to start with? Circle it.]
5. <u>Generate possible obstacles</u>. [What might get in the way of this working? List below.]

6. <u>Address each obstacle</u>. [If you *can't* solve each obstacle, pick a new solution; re-start with #5]
7. <u>Decide on the assignment and do it</u>. [List below exactly when/how you'll do it; then do it!]

8. <u>Evaluate the outcome</u>. [Did it work? If it needs some changes, list them below & try again]

APPENDIX C

HAPPINESS SCALE[1]

This scale is intended to estimate your *current* happiness with your life in each of the 10 areas listed below. Ask yourself the following question as you rate each area:

How happy am I with this area of my life?

Circle one of the numbers (1-10) beside each area. Numbers toward the left indicate various degrees of unhappiness, and numbers toward the right reflect various levels of happiness. In other words, state exactly how you feel today, using the numerical scale (1-10).

Remember: Try to exclude all feelings of yesterday and concentrate only on your feelings *today* in each of these areas. Also, try not to allow one category to influence your answers in the other categories.

	Completely Unhappy						Completely Happy			
Drinking/Drug Use	1	2	3	4	5	6	7	8	9	10
Job or Education Progress	1	2	3	4	5	6	7	8	9	10
Money Management	1	2	3	4	5	6	7	8	9	10
Social Life	1	2	3	4	5	6	7	8	9	10
Personal Habits	1	2	3	4	5	6	7	8	9	10
Marriage/Family Relationships	1	2	3	4	5	6	7	8	9	10
Legal Issues	1	2	3	4	5	6	7	8	9	10
Emotional Life	1	2	3	4	5	6	7	8	9	10
Communication	1	2	3	4	5	6	7	8	9	10
General Happiness	1	2	3	4	5	6	7	8	9	10

[1]*Source: Motivating Substance Abusers to Enter Treatment: Working with Family Members* (p. 223) by J. E. Smith & R. J. Meyers, 2004, New York: Guilford Press. [Copyright by Guilford Press. Adapted by permission.]

Behavioral Couples Therapy
for Alcoholism and Other Drug Abuse

Timothy J. O'Farrell, PhD
William Fals-Stewart, PhD

SUMMARY. Behavioral Couples Therapy (BCT) is designed for married or cohabiting individuals seeking help for alcohol or other drug abuse. BCT sees the drug abusing patient together with the spouse or live-in partner. Its purposes are to build support for abstinence and to improve relationship functioning. BCT promotes abstinence with a

---

Timothy J. O'Farrell is affiliated with the Families and Addiction Program, Department of Psychiatry, Harvard Medical School, and VA Boston Healthcare System, Brockton, MA.

William Fals-Stewart is affiliated with the Department of Psychiatry, University of Rochester School of Medicine, Rochester, NY.

Address correspondence to: Timothy J. O'Farrell, Harvard Medical School Dept. of Psychiatry, VAMC (116B1) - 940 Belmont Street, Brockton, MA 02301 (E-mail: timothy_ofarrell@hms.harvard.edu).

Preparation of this article also was supported by a grant from the National Institute on Alcohol Abuse and Alcoholism (K02AA00234) and by the Department of Veterans Affairs.

This article is adapted from a clinical guideline the authors developed for the Behavioral Health Recovery Management project, a project of Fayette Companies, Peoria, IL and Chestnut Health Systems, Bloomington, IL, that was funded by the Illinois Department of Human Services' Office of Alcoholism and Substance Abuse. This article also draws heavily from the book *Behavioral Couples Therapy for Alcoholism and Drug Abuse* by T. J. O'Farrell and W. Fals-Stewart, copyright 2006 by Guilford Press. Material is used with permission from Fayette Companies and from Guilford Press.

[Haworth co-indexing entry note]: "Behavioral Couples Therapy for Alcoholism and Other Drug Abuse." O'Farrell, Timothy J., and William Fals-Stewart. Co-published simultaneously in *Alcoholism Treatment Quarterly* (The Haworth Press) Vol. 26, No. 1/2, 2008, pp. 195-219; and: *Family Intervention in Substance Abuse: Current Best Practices* (ed: Oliver J. Morgan, and Cheryl H. Litzke) The Haworth Press, 2008, pp. 195-219. Single or multiple copies of this article are available for a fee from The Haworth Document Delivery Service [1-800-HAWORTH, 9:00 a.m. - 5:00 p.m. (EST). E-mail address: docdelivery@haworthpress.com].

Available online at http://atq.haworthpress.com
doi:10.1300/J020v26n01_10

"recovery contract" that involves both members of the couple in a daily ritual to reward abstinence. BCT improves the relationship with techniques for increasing positive activities and improving communication. BCT also fits well with 12-step or other self-help groups, individual or group substance abuse counseling, and recovery medications. doi:10.1300/ J020v26n01_10

KEYWORDS. Alcohol-other drug abuse, behavioral couples therapy, recovery contract

INTRODUCTION

The purpose of Behavioral Couples Therapy (BCT) is to build support for abstinence and to improve relationship functioning among married or cohabiting individuals seeking help for alcoholism or drug abuse. BCT sees the substance abusing patient with the spouse or live-in partner to arrange a daily "Recovery Contract" in which the patient states his or her intent not to drink or use drugs and the spouse expresses support for the patient's efforts to stay abstinent. For patients taking a recovery-related medication (e.g., disulfiram, naltrexone), daily medication ingestion witnessed and verbally reinforced by the spouse also is part of the contract. Self-help meetings and drug urine screens are part of the contract for most patients. BCT also increases positive activities and teaches communication skills.

Research shows that BCT produces greater abstinence and better relationship functioning than typical individual-based treatment and reduces social costs, domestic violence, and emotional problems of the couple's children. Despite the strong evidence base supporting BCT, it is rarely used in substance abuse treatment programs. Low use of BCT may stem from the recency of studies on BCT, many of which were published in the past 15 years. Further, BCT clinical methods and the research supporting BCT have not been widely disseminated. This article will acquaint substance abuse treatment program administrators and clinicians with BCT. Hopefully this will lead to increased use of BCT to the benefit of substance abusing patients and their families. For a more detailed consideration of the material covered in this article, see O'Farrell and Fals-Stewart (2006).

CLINICAL PROCEDURES FOR BEHAVIORAL COUPLES THERAPY

BCT works directly to increase relationship factors conducive to abstinence. A behavioral approach assumes that family members can reward abstinence–and that alcoholic and drug abusing patients from happier, more cohesive relationships with better communication have a lower risk of relapse. The substance abusing patient and the spouse are seen together in BCT, typically for 12-20 weekly outpatient couple sessions over a 3-6 month period. BCT can be an adjunct to individual counseling or it can be the only substance abuse counseling the patient receives. Generally couples are married or cohabiting for at least a year, without current psychosis, and one member of the couple has a current problem with alcoholism and/or drug abuse. The couple starts BCT soon after the substance abuser seeks help. BCT can start immediately after detoxification or a short-term intensive rehab program or when the substance abuser seeks outpatient counseling. The remainder of this section on clinical procedures for BCT is written in the form of instructions to a counselor who wants to use BCT. Table 1 notes key aspects of BCT.

To engage the spouse and the patient together in BCT, first get the substance abusing patient's permission to contact the spouse. Then talk directly to the spouse to invite him or her for an initial BCT couple session. The initial BCT session involves assessing substance abuse and relationship functioning, and then gaining commitment to and starting BCT. You start first with *substance-focused interventions* that continue throughout BCT to promote abstinence. When abstinence and attendance at BCT sessions have stabilized for a few weeks, you add *relationship-focused interventions* to increase positive activities and teach communication. These specific BCT interventions are described in detail next.

TABLE 1. BCT for Alcoholism and Drug Abuse

- The purpose of BCT is to support abstinence and improve relationship functioning.
- The Recovery Contract supports abstinence.
- BCT increases positive activities and improves communication.
- BCT fits well with self-help groups, recovery medications, and other counseling.

Substance-Focused Interventions in BCT

Daily Recovery Contract

You can arrange what we call a daily Recovery Contract. The first part of the contract is the "trust discussion." In it, the patient states his or her intent not to drink or use drugs that day (in the tradition of one day at a time) and the spouse expresses support for the patient's efforts to stay abstinent. For patients taking a recovery-related medication (e.g., disulfiram, naltrexone), daily medication ingestion witnessed and verbally reinforced by the spouse also is part of the contract. The spouse records the performance of the daily contract on a calendar you give him or her. Both partners agree not to discuss past drinking or fears about future drinking at home to prevent substance-related conflicts which can trigger relapse, reserving these discussions for the therapy sessions. At the start of each BCT session, review the Recovery Contract calendar to see how well each spouse has done their part. Have the couple practice their trust discussion (and medication taking if applicable) in each session to highlight its importance and to let you see how they do it. Twelve-step or other self-help meetings are a routine part of BCT for all patients who are willing. Urine drug screens taken at each BCT session are included in BCT for all patients with a current drug problem. If the Recovery Contract includes 12-step meetings or urine drug screens, these are also marked on the calendar and reviewed. The calendar provides an ongoing record of progress that you reward verbally at each session. Table 2 summarizes the components of the Recovery Contract.

Recovery Contract Case Example #1. Figure 1 presents the Recovery Contract and calendar for Mary Smith and her husband Jack. Mary was a 34-year old teacher's aide in an elementary school who had a serious drinking problem and also smoked marijuana daily. She was admitted to a detoxification unit at a community hospital after being caught drinking at work and being suspended from her job. Her husband Jack worked in a local warehouse and was a light drinker with no drug involvement. Mary and Jack had been married 8 years, and Jack was considering leaving the marriage, when the staff at the detoxification unit referred them to the BCT program.

The therapist developed a Recovery Contract in which Mary agreed to a daily "trust discussion" in which she stated to Jack her intent to stay "clean and sober" for the next 24 hours and Jack thanked her for her commitment to sobriety. The couple practiced this ritual in the therapist's

TABLE 2. COMPONENTS OF RECOVERY CONTRACT

- Daily Trust Discussion
  - Alcohol/drug abuser states intention to stay abstinent *that day*
  - Spouse thanks alcohol/drug abuser for efforts to stay abstinent
  - Patient thanks spouse for support
  - Couple does not argue about past or future substance use
- Medication to aid recovery
- Self-help involvement
- Weekly urine drug screens
- Other weekly activities to support recovery
- Progress recorded on calendar

office until it felt comfortable, and then also performed the discussion at each weekly therapy session on Wednesday evening. As the calendar in Figure 1 shows, they did this part of the contract nearly every day, missing only on an occasional Saturday because their schedule was different that day and sometimes they forgot. Mary agreed to at least 2 AA meetings each week and actually attended 3 meetings per week for the first two months. Jack was pleased to see Mary not drinking and going to AA. However, he was upset that weekly drug urine screens were positive for marijuana for the first few weeks, taking this as evidence that his wife was still smoking marijuana even though she denied it. The therapist explained that marijuana could stay in the system for some time particularly in someone who had been a daily pot smoker. The therapist suggested Jack go to Al-Anon to help him deal with his distress over his wife's suspected drug use. After a few weeks, the drug screens were negative for marijuana and stayed that way lending further credence to Mary's daily statement of intent. Jack found Al-Anon helpful and the couple added to their contract that one night a week they would go together to a local church where Mary could attend an AA meeting and Jack an Al-Anon meeting.

Recovery Contract with a Recovery Medication

A medication to aid recovery is often part of BCT. Medications include Naltrexone for heroin-addicted or alcoholic patients and Antabuse (disulfiram) for alcoholic patients. Antabuse is a drug that produces extreme nausea and sickness when the person taking it drinks. As such it is an option for drinkers with a goal of abstinence. Traditional Antabuse therapy often is not effective because the drinker stops taking it. The Antabuse Contract, also part of the Community Reinforcement Approach,

FIGURE 1
Recovery Contract

In order to help (patient) _____**Mary**_____ with his/her recovery and to bring peace of mind to

(partner) _____**Jack**_____, we commit to the following:

Patient's Responsibilities	Partner's Responsibilities
☒ DAILY TRUST DISCUSSION (with medication **N.A.** if taking it)	
• States his/her intention to stay substance free that day (and takes medication if applicable).	• Records that the intention was shared (and medication taken if applicable) on calendar.
• Thanks partner for supporting his/her recovery.	• Thanks patient for his/her recovery efforts.
☒ FOCUS ON PRESENT AND FUTURE, NOT PAST	
• If necessary, requests that partner not mention past or possible future substance abuse outside of counseling sessions.	• Agrees not to mention past substance abuse or fears of future substance abuse outside of counseling sessions.
☒ WEEKLY SELF-HELP MEETINGS	
• Commitment to 12-Step mtgs: **AA mtgs 7pm Tues at church 10am Sat at hospital**	• Commitment to 12-Step mtgs: **Al-Anon mtg 7pm Tues at church**
☒ URINE DRUG SCREENS	
• Urine Drug Screens: **Weekly at counseling sessions**	
☐ OTHER RECOVERY SUPPORT	
• _____	• _____

EARLY WARNING SYSTEM
If, at any time the trust discussion (with medication if taking it) does not take place for two days in a row, we will contact (therapist/phone #: **Dr. Tim O'Farrell   123-456-7899**) immediately.

LENGTH OF CONTRACT
This agreement covers the time from today until the end of weekly therapy sessions, when it can be renewed. It cannot be changed unless all of those signing below discuss the changes together.

Mary Smith
Patient

Tim O'Farrell Ph. D.
Therapist

Jack Smith
Partner

9 / **12** / **xx**
Date

FIGURE 1 (Continued)
Recovery Contract Calendar

☒ ✓ = Trust Discussion Done

☐ (✓) = Trust Discussion with Medication (_____)

☒ A = AA or NA meeting

☒ N = Alanon or Naranon

☒ D = Drug Urine + or −

☐ O = Other (_____

September						
S	M	T	W	T	F	S
						1
2	3	4	✓ D+ 5	✓ 6	✓ 7	8
✓ 9	✓ A 10	✓ 11	✓ D+ 12	✓ 13	✓ A 14	✓ 15
✓ 16	✓ 17	✓ A 18	✓ D+ 19	✓ 20	✓ A 21	✓ A 22
✓ 23	✓ A N 24	✓ 25	✓ D− 26	✓ 27	✓ A 28	✓ A 29
✓ 30						

October						
S	M	T	W	T	F	S
				✓ 1	✓ A N 2	✓ D− 3	✓ 4	✓ 5	✓ A 6
✓ 7	✓ A N 8	✓ 9	✓ D− 10	✓ 11	✓ A 12	✓ A 13
✓ 14	✓ 15	✓ 16	✓ D− 17	✓ 18	✓ A 19	✓ A 20
✓ 21	✓ 22	✓ A N 23	✓ D− 24	✓ 25	✓ A 26	✓ A 27
✓ 28	✓ 29	✓ A N 30	✓ D− 31			

November						
S	M	T	W	T	F	S
				✓ 1	✓ 2	✓ A 3
✓ 4	✓ 5	✓ A N 6	✓ D− 7	✓ 8	✓ 9	A 10
✓ 11	✓ 12	✓ A N 13	✓ D− 14	✓ 15	✓ 16	✓ A 17
✓ 18	✓ 19	✓ A N 20	✓ D− 21	✓ 22	✓ 23	24
✓ 25	✓ 26	✓ A N 27	✓ D− 28	✓ 29	✓ 30	

December						
S	M	T	W	T	F	S
						✓ A 1
✓ 2	✓ 3	✓ A 4	✓ D− 5	✓ 6	✓ 7	✓ A 8
✓ 9	✓ 10	✓ A N 11	✓ D− 12	✓ 13	✓ 14	✓ A 15
✓ 16	✓ 17	✓ A N 18	✓ D− 19	✓ 20	✓ 21	✓ A 22
✓ 23	✓ 24	✓ 25	✓ 26	✓ 27	✓ 28	✓ A 29
✓ 30	✓ 31					

significantly improves compliance in taking the medication and increases abstinence rates. In the Antabuse Contract, the drinker agrees to take Antabuse each day while the spouse observes. The spouse, in turn, agrees to positively reinforce the drinker for taking the Antabuse, to record the observation on a calendar you provide them, and not to mention past drinking or any fears about future drinking. Each spouse should view the agreement as a cooperative method for rebuilding lost trust and not as a coercive checking-up operation. Before negotiating such a contract, make sure that the drinker is willing and medically cleared to take Antabuse and that both the drinker and spouse have been fully informed and educated about the effects of the drug. This is done by the prescribing physician but double check their level of understanding about it.

Recovery Contract Case Example #2. Figure 2 presents the Recovery Contract and calendar for Bill Jones, a 42-year old truck driver with a chronic alcoholism problem, and his wife Nancy who drank only occasionally. The staff at the detoxification unit also referred this couple to our program. Daily Antabuse observed and reinforced by the wife was part of their contract in addition to the daily trust discussion in which Bill stated his intent to stay sober. Drug urine screens were not part of the contract because Bill did not have a problem with any substance other than alcohol. The therapist thought each member of the couple was a good candidate to benefit from 12-step meetings, but Bill refused AA and Nancy was reluctant to attend Al-Anon. Thus, 12-step meetings were not part of their contract. During the first 2 weeks of trying out the contract, they were inconsistent in performing the contract due to logistical problems and to their continued anger and distrust with each other–a common problem. The therapist worked with the couple to overcome these problems and the couple eventually did the contract consistently each day and felt they benefitted from it. After 6 months Bill stopped taking Antabuse, but the daily trust discussion was continued for an additional 6 months and this proved a satisfactory arrangement for both Bill and Nancy.

Other Support for Abstinence

Reviewing urges to drink or use drugs experienced in the past week is part of each BCT session. This includes thoughts and temptations that are less intense than an urge or a craving. Discussing situations, thoughts and feelings associated with urges helps identify potential triggers or cues for alcohol or drug use. It can help alert you to the possible risk of a

FIGURE 2
Recovery Contract

In order to help (patient) __**Bill**__ with his/her recovery and to bring peace of mind to (partner) __**Nancy**__, we commit to the following:

Patient's Responsibilities	Partner's Responsibilities
☒ DAILY TRUST DISCUSSION (with medication **Antabuse** if taking it)	
• States his/her intention to stay substance free that day (and takes medication if applicable).	• Records that the intention was shared (and medication taken if applicable) on calendar.
• Thanks partner for supporting his/her recovery.	• Thanks patient for his/her recovery efforts.
☒ FOCUS ON PRESENT AND FUTURE, NOT PAST	
• If necessary, requests that partner not mention past or possible future substance abuse outside of counseling sessions.	• Agrees not to mention past substance abuse or fears of future substance abuse outside of counseling sessions.
☐ WEEKLY SELF-HELP MEETINGS	
• Commitment to 12-Step mtgs:_____	• Commitment to 12-Step mtgs:_____
☐ URINE DRUG SCREENS	
• Urine Drug Screens: _____	
☐ OTHER RECOVERY SUPPORT	
• _____	• _____

EARLY WARNING SYSTEM
If, at any time the trust discussion (with medication if taking it) does not take place for two days in a row, we will contact (therapist/phone #: __**Dr. Tim O'Farrell 123-456-7899**__) immediately.

LENGTH OF CONTRACT
This agreement covers the time from today until the end of weekly therapy sessions, when it can be renewed. It cannot be changed unless all of those signing below discuss the changes together.

**Bill Jones**
Patient

**Tim O'Farrell Ph.D**
Therapist

**Nancy Jones**
Partner

__**9** / **13** / **XX**__
Date

FIGURE 2 (Continued)
Recovery Contract

☐ ✓ = **Trust Discussion Done**   ☐ **N = Alanon or Naranon**

☒ (✓) = **Trust Discussion with**   ☐ **D = Drug Urine + or −**
              Medication (Antabuse)

☐ **A = AA or NA meeting**   ☐ **O = Other (_____)**

	September								October					
S	**M**	**T**	**W**	**T**	**F**	**S**	**S**	**M**	**T**	**W**	**T**	**F**	**S**
						1	① 1	① 2	① 3	① 4	① 5	① 6	
2	3	4	5	① 6	7	① 8	① 7	① 8	① 9	① 10	① 11	① 12	① 13
① 9	① 10	① 11	12	① 13	14	① 15	14	① 15	① 16	① 17	① 18	① 19	① 20
① 16	17	① 18	19	① 20	① 21	① 22	① 21	① 22	① 23	① 24	25	26	① 27
23	① 24	① 25	① 26	① 27	① 28	29	① 28	① 29	① 30	① 31			
① 30													

	November								December					
S	**M**	**T**	**W**	**T**	**F**	**S**	**S**	**M**	**T**	**W**	**T**	**F**	**S**
				① 1	① 2	① 3							① 1
① 4	① 5	① 6	① 7	① 8	① 9	① 10	① 2	① 3	4	① 5	① 6	① 7	① 8
① 11	① 12	① 13	① 14	① 15	① 16	① 17	① 9	10	① 11	① 12	① 13	① 14	① 15
① 18	19	① 20	① 21	✓ 22	① 23	① 24	① 16	① 17	① 18	① 19	① 20	① 21	① 22
① 25	26	① 27	① 28	① 29	① 30		① 23	① 24	① 25	① 26	① 27	① 28	① 29
							① 30	① 31					

relapse. It also identifies successful coping strategies (e.g., distraction, calling a sponsor) the patient used to resist an urge, and it builds confidence for the future.

Crisis intervention for substance use is an important part of BCT. Drinking or drug use episodes occur during BCT as with any other treatment. BCT works best if you intervene before the substance use goes on for too long a period. In an early BCT session, negotiate an agreement that either member of the couple should call you if substance use occurs or if they fear it is imminent. Once substance use has occurred, try to get it stopped and see the couple as soon as possible to use the relapse as a learning experience. At the couple session, you must be extremely active in defusing hostile or depressive reactions to the substance use. Stress that drinking or drug use does not constitute total failure, that inconsistent progress is the rule rather than the exception. Help the couple decide what they need to do to feel sure that the substance use is over and will not continue in the coming week (e.g., restarting recovery medication, going to AA and Al-Anon together, reinstituting a daily Recovery Contract, entering a detoxification unit). Finally, try to help the couple identify what triggers led up to the relapse and generate alternative solutions other than substance use for similar future situations.

Relationship-Focused Interventions in BCT

Once the Recovery Contract is going smoothly, the substance abuser has been abstinent and the couple has been keeping scheduled appointments for a few weeks, you can start to focus on improving couple and family relationships. Family members often experience resentment about past substance abuse and fear and distrust about the possible return of substance abuse in the future. The substance abuser often experiences guilt and a desire for recognition of current improved behavior. These feelings experienced by the substance abuser and the family often lead to an atmosphere of tension and unhappiness in couple and family relationships. There are problems caused by substance use (e.g., bills, legal charges, embarrassing incidents) that still need to be resolved. There is often a backlog of other unresolved couple and family problems that the substance use obscured. The couple frequently lacks the mutual positive feelings and communication skills needed to resolve these problems. As a result, many marriages and families are dissolved during the first 1 or 2 years of the substance abuser's recovery. In other cases, couple and family conflicts trigger relapse and a return to substance abuse. Even in cases where the substance abuser has a basically sound marriage and family life when he or she is not abusing substances, the initiation of abstinence can produce temporary tension and role readjustment and provide the opportunity for stabilizing and enriching couple and family relationships. For these reasons, many substance abusing patients can benefit from assistance to improve their couple and family relationships.

Two major goals of interventions focused on the substance abuser's couple relationship are (a) to increase positive feeling, goodwill, and commitment to the relationship; and (b) to teach communication skills to resolve conflicts, problems, and desires for change. The general sequence in teaching couples and families skills to increase positive activities and improve communication is (a) therapist instruction and modeling, (b) the couple practicing under your supervision, (c) assignment for homework, and (d) review of homework with further practice. Table 3 summarizes relationship-focused interventions in BCT.

Increasing Positive Activities

Catch Your Partner Doing Something Nice. A series of procedures can increase a couple's awareness of benefits from the relationship and the frequency with which spouses notice, acknowledge, and initiate pleasing or caring behaviors on a daily basis. Tell the couple that caring behaviors are "behaviors showing that you care for the other person," and assign homework called "Catch Your Partner Doing Something Nice" to assist couples in noticing daily caring behaviors. This requires each spouse to record one caring behavior performed by the partner each day on sheets you provide them (see Figure 3). The couple reads the caring behaviors recorded during the previous week at the subsequent session. Then you model acknowledging caring behaviors ("I liked it when you . . . It made me feel _____ ."), noting the importance of eye contact; a smile;

TABLE 3. Relationship-Focused Interventions in BCT

- Increasing Positive Activities
  - Catch Your Partner Doing Something Nice
  - Caring Day Assignment
  - Shared Rewarding Activities
- Teaching Communication
  - Listening Skills
  - Expressing Feelings Directly
  - Communication Sessions
  - Negotiating for Requests

FIGURE 3.
Catch Your Partner Doing Something Nice

Each day, notice at least one nice thing that your partner does and note it on the following chart. It is ALWAYS POSSIBLE to notice at least one CARING BEHAVIOR–even if you do not see your partner for an entire day. Don't share your list with your partner yet!

Day	Date	Caring Behavior
Monday	4/6	Waited to have dinner with me because I had to stay late at work. Made me feel good.
Tues	4/7	Told me she loved me.
Wed	4/8	Cooked a delicious Italian dinner and afterwards we had a very romantic evening.
Thurs	4/9	Was patient with me as I came home tired and moody from work.
Friday	4/10	Enjoyed a walk together around the neighborhood.
Sat	4/11	Woke me gently and rubbed my back.
Sun	4/12	She asked me how my day was and listened to me talk.

a sincere, pleasant tone of voice; and only positive feelings. Each spouse then practices acknowledging caring behaviors from his or her daily list for the previous week.

After the couple practices the new behavior in the therapy session, assign for homework a 2-5 minute daily communication session at home in which each partner acknowledges one pleasing behavior noticed that day. These daily brief acknowledgments often are done at the same time as the "trust discussion" that is part of the Recovery Contract. As couples begin to notice and acknowledge daily caring behaviors, each partner begins initiating more caring behaviors. Often the weekly reports of daily caring behaviors show that one or both spouses are fulfilling requests for desired change voiced before the therapy. In addition, many couples report that the 2-5 minute communication sessions result in more extensive conversations.

Planning Shared Rewarding Activities. Many substance abusers' families stop shared recreational and leisure activities due to strained relationships and embarrassing substance-related incidents. Reversing this trend is important because participation by the couple and family in social and recreational activities improves substance abuse treatment outcomes (Moos, Finney, & Cronkite, 1990). Planning and engaging in shared rewarding activities can be started by simply having each spouse make a separate list of possible activities. Each activity must involve both spouses, either by themselves or with their children or other adults and can be at or away from home. Before giving the couple homework of planning a shared activity, model planning an activity to illustrate solutions to common pitfalls (e.g., waiting until the last minute so that necessary preparations cannot be made, getting sidetracked on trivial practical arrangements). Finally, instruct the couple to refrain from discussing problems or conflicts during their planned activity.

Caring Day. A final assignment is that each partner give the other a "Caring Day" during the coming week by performing special acts to show caring for the spouse. Encourage each partner to take risks and to act lovingly toward the spouse rather than wait for the other to make the first move. Finally, remind spouses that at the start of therapy they agreed to act differently (e.g., more lovingly) and then assess changes in feelings, rather than wait to feel more positively toward their partner before instituting changes in their own behavior.

Teaching Communication Skills

We generally begin our work on training in communication skills by defining effective communication as "message intended (by speaker) equals message received (by listener)" and emphasizing the need to learn both "listening" and "speaking" skills. The chart presented in Figure 4 helps expand this definition further including factors (e.g., "filters") in each person that can impede communication.

FIGURE 4. Message Intended = Message Received

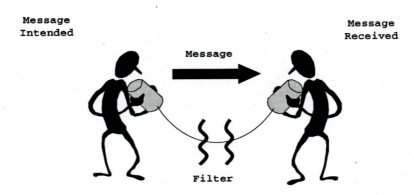

Teaching couples communication skills of listening and speaking and how to use planned communication sessions are essential prerequisites for negotiating desired behavior changes. Start this training with non-problem areas that are positive or neutral and move to problem areas and emotionally charged issues only after each skill has been practiced on easier topics.

Listening Skills. Good listening helps each spouse to feel understood and supported and to slow down couple interactions to prevent quick escalation of aversive exchanges. Instruct spouses to repeat both the words and the feelings of the speaker's message and to check to see if the message they received was the message intended by their partner ("What I heard you say was . . . Is that right?"). When the listener has understood the speaker's message, roles change and the first listener then speaks. Teaching a partner to communicate support and understanding by summarizing the spouse's message and checking the accuracy of the received message before stating his or her own position is often a major accomplishment that has to be achieved gradually. A partner's failure to separate understanding the spouse's position from agreement with it often is an obstacle that must be overcome.

Expressing Feelings Directly. Expressing both positive and negative feelings directly is an alternative to the blaming, hostile, and indirect responsibility-avoiding communication behaviors that characterize many substance abusers' relationships. Emphasize that when the speaker expresses feelings directly, there is a greater chance that he or she will be heard because the speaker says these are his or her feelings, his or her point of view, and not some objective fact about the other person. The speaker takes responsibility for his or her own feelings and does not blame the other person for how he or she feels. This reduces listener defensiveness and makes it easier for the listener to receive the intended message. Present examples of differences between direct expressions of feelings and indirect and ineffective or hurtful expressions. The use of statements beginning with "I" rather than "you" is emphasized. After presenting the rationale and instructions, model correct and incorrect ways of expressing feelings and elicit the couple's reactions to these modeled scenes. Then have the couple role-play a communication session in which spouses take turns being speaker and listener, with the speaker expressing feelings directly and the listener using the listening response. During this role-playing, coach the couple as they practice reflecting the direct expressions of feelings. Assign for homework similar communication sessions, 10 to 15 minutes each, three to four times weekly. Subsequent therapy sessions involve more practice with role-playing, both during the sessions and for homework. Increase in difficulty each week the topics on which the couple practices.

Communication Sessions. These are planned, structured discussions in which spouses talk privately, face-to-face, without distractions, and with each spouse taking turns expressing his or her point of view without interruptions. Communication sessions can be introduced for 2-5 minutes daily when couples first practice acknowledging caring behaviors. In later weeks when the couple discusses current relationship problems or concerns, communication sessions typically are assigned for 10- to 15-minutes three to four times a week. Discuss with the couple the time and place that they plan to have their assigned communication practice sessions. Assess the success of this plan at the next session, and suggest any needed changes. Just establishing a communication session as a method for discussing feelings, events, and problems can be very helpful for many couples. Encourage couples to ask each other for a communication session when they want to discuss an issue or problem, keeping in mind the ground rules of behavior that characterize such a session.

Negotiating for Requests. Many changes that spouses desire from their partners can be achieved through the caring behaviors, rewarding activities, and communication skills that have already been mentioned. However, deeper, emotion-laden conflicts that have caused considerable hostility and arguments for years are more resistant to change. Learning to make positive specific requests and to negotiate and compromise can lead to agreements to resolve such issues.

Positive specific requests are an alternative to the all-too-frequent practice of couples complaining in vague and unclear terms and trying to coerce, browbeat, and force the other partner to change. For homework each partner lists at least five requests. Negotiation and compromise comes next. Spouses share their lists of requests, starting with the most specific and positive items. Give feedback on the requests presented and help rewrite items as needed. Then explain that negotiating and compromising can help couples reach an agreement in which each partner will do one thing requested by the other. After giving instructions and examples, coach a couple while they have a communication session in which requests are made in a positive specific form, heard by each partner, and translated into a mutually satisfactory, realistic agreement for the upcoming week. Finally, record the agreement on a homework sheet that the couple knows you will review with them during the next session. Such agreements can be a major focus of a number of BCT sessions.

Maintenance and Relapse Prevention

We suggest using three general methods to promote long-term maintenance of the changes in substance problems made through BCT. First, plan maintenance prior to the termination of the weekly treatment phase. This involves helping the couple complete a Continuing Recovery Plan that specifies which behaviors from the previous BCT sessions they wish to continue (e.g., daily trust discussion, AA meetings, shared rewarding activities, communication sessions). Second, anticipate high-risk situations for relapse that may occur after weekly treatment ends. Discuss and rehearse possible coping strategies that the substance abuser and spouse can use to prevent relapse when confronted with such situations. Third, discuss and rehearse how to cope with a relapse if it occurs. A specific relapse plan, written and rehearsed prior to ending weekly treatment, can be particularly useful. Early intervention at the beginning of a relapse episode is essential: impress the couple with this point. Often, individuals wait until the substance use has reached dangerous levels again before acting. By then, much additional damage has been done to couple and family relationships and to other aspects of the substance abuser's life.

We suggest continued contact with the couple via planned in-person and telephone follow-up sessions, at regular and then gradually increasing intervals, preferably for 3 to 5 years after a stable pattern of recovery has been achieved. Use this ongoing contact to monitor progress, to assess compliance with the Continuing Recovery Plan, and to evaluate the need for additional therapy sessions. You must take responsibility for scheduling and reminding the couple of follow-up sessions and for placing agreed-upon phone calls so that continued contact can be maintained successfully. Tell couples the reason for continued contact is that substance abuse is a chronic health problem that requires active, aggressive, ongoing monitoring to prevent or to quickly treat relapses for at least 5 years after an initial stable pattern of recovery has been established. The follow-up contact also provides the opportunity to deal with couple and family issues that appear after a period of recovery.

Contraindications for BCT

A few contraindications for BCT should be considered. First, couples in which there is a court-issued restraining order for the spouses not to have contact with each other should not be seen together in therapy until the restraining order is lifted or modified to allow contact in counseling.

Second, couples are excluded from BCT if very severe domestic violence (defined as resulting in injury requiring medical attention or hospitalization) has occurred in the past two years or if one or both members of the couple fear that taking part in couples treatment may stimulate violence (Fals-Stewart & Kennedy, 2005; O'Farrell & Fals-Stewart, 2006). Although domestic violence is quite common among substance abuse patients, most of this violence is not so severe that it precludes BCT. In our experience fewer than 2% of couples seeking BCT are excluded from being treated in BCT due to very severe violence or fears of couples therapy. The best plan in the vast majority of cases is to address the violence in BCT sessions by teaching a commitment to nonviolence, communication skills to reduce hostile conflicts, and coping skills to minimize conflict if the substance abuser relapses (for more details see O'Farrell & Fals-Stewart, 2006; O'Farrell & Murphy, 2002). Research reviewed below shows that violence is substantially reduced after BCT and virtually eliminated for patients who stay abstinent.

Finally, if the spouse also has a current alcohol or drug problem, BCT may not be effective. In the past, we have often taken the stance that if both members of a couple have a substance use problem, then we will not treat them together unless one member of the couple has at least 90 days abstinence. However, in a recent project we successfully treated couples in which both the male and female partner had a current alcoholism problem (Schumm, O'Farrell, Murphy, & Fals-Stewart, 2006). If both members of the couple want to stop drinking or if this mutual decision to change can be reached in the first few sessions, then BCT may be workable.

EFFECTIVENESS OF BEHAVIORAL COUPLES THERAPY

Meta-analytic reviews of randomized studies show more abstinence with family-involved treatment than with individual treatment in drug abuse (Stanton & Shadish, 1997) and in alcoholism (O'Farrell & Fals-Stewart, 2001). Overall the effect size favoring family-involved treatments over individual-based treatments was classified as a medium-size effect. This effect size is 10 times greater than that observed for aspirin in preventing heart attacks, an effect considered important in medical research (Rosenthal, 1991). BCT is the family therapy method with the strongest research support for its effectiveness in substance abuse (Epstein & McCrady, 1998). Table 4 summarizes results of studies on BCT that are covered below.

TABLE 4. Studies of BCT Show

- BCT produces more abstinence, happier relationships, and fewer separations than individual treatment
- Benefit to cost ratio for BCT is greater than 5 to1
- Domestic violence is greatly reduced in BCT
- BCT helps a couple's children more than individual treatment for a parent
- BCT improves compliance with recovery medications (e.g., disulfiram, naltrexone)
- Evidence supports wider use of BCT

Primary Clinical Outcomes: Abstinence and Relationship Functioning

A series of studies have compared substance abuse and relationship outcomes for substance abusing patients treated with BCT or individual counseling. Outcomes have been measured at 6-months follow-up in earlier studies and at 12-24 months after treatment in more recent studies. The studies show a fairly consistent pattern of more abstinence and fewer substance-related problems, happier relationships, and lower risk of couple separation and divorce for substance abusing patients who receive BCT than for patients who receive only more typical individual-based treatment. These results come from studies with mostly male alcoholic (Azrin, Sisson, Meyers, & Godley, 1982; Bowers & Al-Rehda, 1990; Chick et al., 1992; Hedberg & Campbell, 1974; Fals-Stewart, Klosterman, Yates, O'Farrell, & Birchler, 2005; Fals-Stewart & O'Farrell, 2002; Kelley & Fals-Stewart, 2002; McCrady, Stout, Noel, Abrams, & Nelson, 1991; O'Farrell, Cutter, Choquette, Floyd, & Bayog, 1992) and drug abusing (Fals-Stewart, Birchler & O'Farrell, 1996; Fals-Stewart & O'Farrell, 2003; Fals-Stewart, O'Farrell, & Birchler, 2001a, 2001b; Kelley & Fals-Stewart, 2002) patients and also with female alcoholic (Fals-Stewart, Birchler, & Kelley, 2006) and drug abusing patients (Winters, Fals-Stewart, O'Farrell, Birchler, & Kelley, 2002).

Social Cost Outcomes and Benefit-to-Cost Ratio

Three studies (2 in alcoholism and 1 in drug abuse) have examined social cost outcomes after BCT (O'Farrell et al., 1996a, 1996b; Fals-Stewart, O'Farrell, & Birchler, 1997). These social costs included costs for substance abuse-related health care, criminal justice system use for substance-related crimes, and income from illegal sources and public assistance. The average social costs per case decreased substantially in the 1-2 years after as compared to the year before BCT, with cost savings averaging $5,000-$6,500 per case. Reduced social costs after BCT saved more than 5 times the cost of delivering BCT, producing a benefit-to-cost ratio greater than 5:1. Thus, for every dollar spent in delivering BCT, 5 dollars in social costs are saved. In addition, BCT was more cost-effective when compared with individual treatment for drug abuse (Fals-Stewart et al., 1997) and when compared with interactional couples therapy for alcoholism (O'Farrell et al., 1996b).

Domestic Violence Outcomes

A recent study (O'Farrell, Murphy, Stephan, Fals-Stewart, & Murphy, 2004) examined male-to-female partner violence before and after BCT for 303 married or cohabiting male alcoholic patients. There also was a demographically matched comparison sample of couples without alcohol problems. In the year before BCT, 60% of alcoholic patients had been violent toward their female partner, five times the comparison sample rate of 12%. In the year after BCT, violence decreased significantly to 24% of the alcoholic sample but remained higher than the comparison group. Among remitted alcoholics after BCT, violence prevalence of 12% was identical to the comparison sample and less than half the rate among relapsed patients (30%). Results for the second year after BCT were similar to the first year. An earlier study (O'Farrell & Murphy, 1995) found nearly identical results. Thus, these 2 studies showed that male-to-female violence was significantly reduced in the first and second year after BCT and that it was nearly eliminated with abstinence.

Two recent studies showed that BCT reduced partner violence and couple conflicts better than individual treatment. Among male drug abusing patients, while nearly half of the couples reported male-to-female violence in the year before treatment, the number reporting violence in the year after treatment was significantly lower for BCT (17%) than for individual treatment (42%) (Fals-Stewart, Kashdan, O'Farrell, Birchler, & Kelley, 2002). Among male alcoholic patients, those who participated in BCT reported less frequent use of maladaptive responses to conflict (e.g., yelling, name-calling, threatening to hit, hitting) during treatment than those who received individual treatment (Birchler & Fals-Stewart, 2001). These results suggest that in BCT couples do learn to handle their conflicts with less hostility and aggression.

Impact of BCT on the Children of Couples Undergoing BCT

Kelley and Fals-Stewart (2002) conducted 2 studies (1 in alcoholism, 1 in drug abuse) to find out whether BCT for a substance abusing parent, with its demonstrated reductions in domestic violence and reduced risk for family breakup, also has beneficial effects for the children in the family. Results were the same for children of male alcoholic and male drug abusing fathers. BCT improved children's functioning in the year after the parents' treatment more than did individual-based treatment or couple psychoeducation. Only BCT showed reduction in the number of children with clinically significant impairment.

Integrating BCT with Recovery Related Medication

BCT has been used to increase compliance with a recovery-related medication. Fals-Stewart and O'Farrell (2003) compared BCT with individual treatment for male opioid-addicted patients taking naltrexone. BCT patients, compared with their individually treated counterparts, had better naltrexone compliance, greater abstinence, and fewer substance-related problems. Fals-Stewart, O'Farrell and Martin (2002) found that BCT produced better compliance with HIV medications among HIV-positive drug abusers in an outpatient drug abuse treatment program than did treatment as usual. BCT also has improved compliance with pharmacotherapy in studies of disulfiram for alcoholic patients (e.g., Azrin et al., 1982; Chick et al., 1992; O'Farrell et al., 1992) and in a pilot study of naltrexone with alcoholics (Fals-Stewart & O'Farrell, 2002).

BCT with Family Members Other than Spouses

Most BCT studies have examined traditional couples. However, some recent studies have expanded BCT to include family members other than spouses. These studies have targeted increased medication compliance as just described. For example, in the study of BCT and naltrexone with opioid patients (Fals-Stewart & O'Farrell, 2003), family members taking part were spouses (66%), parents (25%), and siblings (9%). In the study of BCT and HIV medications among HIV-positive drug abusers (Fals-Stewart, O'Farrell & Martin, 2002), significant others who took part were: a parent or sibling (67%), a homosexual (12%) or heterosexual (9%) partner, or a roommate (12%).

Needed Research

In terms of future directions, we do need more research on BCT, to replicate and extend the most recent advances, especially for women patients and broader family constellations. Research on BCT for couples in which both the male and female member have a current substance use problem is particularly needed because prior BCT studies have not addressed this difficult clinical challenge. Even more than additional research, we need technology transfer so that patients and their families can benefit from what we have already learned about BCT for alcoholism and drug abuse.

CONCLUSIONS

The purpose of Behavioral Couples Therapy is to build support for abstinence and to improve relationship functioning among married or cohabiting individuals seeking help for alcoholism or drug abuse. Research shows that BCT produces greater abstinence and better relationship functioning than typical individual-based treatment and reduces social costs, domestic violence, and emotional problems of the couple's children. BCT fits well with 12-step or other self-help groups, individual or group substance abuse counseling, and recovery medications. Thus research evidence supports wider use of BCT. We hope this article will lead to increased use of BCT to the benefit of substance abusing patients and their families. In addition, three new resources are available for those interested in learning more about how to implement BCT:

1. A comprehensive counselor's guide book to implementing BCT O'Farrell, T. J. & Fals-Stewart, W. (2006). *Behavioral couples therapy for alcoholism and drug abuse.* New York: Guilford Press.
2. A website from which BCT therapist manuals and materials can be obtained *www.addictionandfamily.org*
3. A web-based distance learning course on BCT *www.neattc.org/ training.htm*

REFERENCES

Azrin, N. H., Sisson, R. W., Meyers, R., & Godley, M. (1982). Alcoholism treatment by Disulfiram and community reinforcement therapy. *Journal of Behavior Therapy and Experimental Psychiatry, 13*, 105-112.
Birchler, G. R., & Fals-Stewart, W. (2001). *Use of behavioral couples therapy with alcoholic couples: Effects on maladaptive responses to conflict during treatment.*

Poster presented at the 35th Annual Convention of the Association for the Advancement of Behavior Therapy, Philadelphia, PA.

Bowers, T. G., & Al-Rehda, M. R. (1990). A comparison of outcome with group/marital and standard/individual therapies with alcoholics. *Journal of Studies on Alcohol*, *51*, 301-309.

Chick, J., Gough, K., Falkowski, W., Kershaw, P., Hore, B., Mehta, B., Ritson, B., Ropner, R., & Torley, D. (1992). Disulfiram treatment of alcoholism. *British Journal of Psychiatry*, *161*, 84-89.

Epstein, E. E., & McCrady, B. S. (1998). Behavioral couples treatment of alcohol and drug use disorders: Current status and innovations. *Clinical Psychology Review*, *18*, 689-711.

Fals-Stewart, W., Birchler, G. R., & Kelley, M. L. (2006). Learning Sobriety Together: A randomized clinical trial examining behavioral couples therapy with female alcoholic patients. *Journal of Consulting and Clinical Psychology*, *74*, 579-591.

Fals-Stewart, W., Birchler, G. R., & O'Farrell, T. J. (1996). Behavioral couples therapy for male substance-abusing patients: Effects on relationship adjustment and drug-using behavior. *Journal of Consulting and Clinical Psychology*, *64*, 959-972.

Fals-Stewart, W., Kashdan, T. B., O'Farrell, T. J., & Birchler, G. R. (2002). Behavioral couples therapy for male-drug abusing patients and their partners: The effect on interpartner violence. *Journal of Substance Abuse Treatment*, *22*, 1-10.

Fals-Stewart, W., & Kennedy, C. (2005). Addressing intimate partner violence in substance-abuse treatment. *Journal of Substance Abuse Treatment*, *29*, 5-17.

Fals-Stewart, W., Klosterman, K., Yates, B. T., O'Farrell, T. J., & Birchler, G. R. (2005). Brief relationship therapy for alcoholism: A randomized clinical trial examining clinical efficacy and cost-effectiveness. *Psychology of Addictive Behaviors*, *19*, 363-371.

Fals-Stewart, W., & O'Farrell, T. J. (2003). Behavioral family counseling and naltrexone for male opioid dependent patients. *Journal of Consulting and Clinical Psychology*, *71*, 432-442.

Fals-Stewart, W., & O'Farrell, T. J. (2002). *Behavioral couples therapy increases compliance with naltrexone among male alcoholic patients.* Unpublished data. Research institute on Addiction, Buffalo NY.

Fals-Stewart, W., O'Farrell, T. J., & Birchler. G. R. (1997). Behavioral couples therapy for male substance abusing patients: A cost outcomes analysis. *Journal of Consulting and Clinical Psychology*, *65*, 789-802.

Fals-Stewart, W., O'Farrell, T. J., & Birchler, G. R. (2001a). Behavioral couples therapy for male methadone maintenance patients: Effects on drug-using behavior and relationship adjustment. *Behavior Therapy*, *32*, 391-411.

Fals-Stewart, W., O'Farrell, T. J., & Birchler, G. R. (2001b). Use of abbreviated couples therapy in substance abuse. In J. V. Cordova (Chair), *Approaches to Brief Couples Therapy: Application and Efficiency.* Symposium conducted at the World Congress of Behavioral and Cognitive Therapies, Vancouver, Canada.

Fals-Stewart, W., O'Farrell, T. J., & Martin, J. (2002). Using behavioral family counseling to enhance HIV-medication compliance among HIV-infected male drug abusing patients. Paper presented at conference on "Treating Addictions in Special Populations," Binghamton, NY.

Hedberg, A. G., & Campbell, L. (1974). A comparison of four behavioral treatments of alcoholism. *Journal of Behavior Therapy and Experimental Psychiatry, 5,* 251-256.

Kelley, M. L., & Fals-Stewart, W. (2002). Couples versus individual-based therapy for alcoholism and drug abuse: Effects on children's psychosocial functioning. *Journal of Consulting and Clinical Psychology, 70,* 417-427.

McCrady, B., Stout, R., Noel, N., Abrams, D., & Nelson, H. (1991). Comparative effectiveness of three types of spouse involved alcohol treatment: Outcomes 18 months after treatment. *British Journal of Addiction, 86,* 1415-1424.

Moos, R. H., Finney, J. W., & Cronkite, R. C. (1990). *Alcoholism treatment: Context, process, and outcome.* New York: Oxford University Press.

O'Farrell, T. J., Choquette, K. A., Cutter, H. S. G., Floyd, F. J., Bayog, R. D., Brown, E. D., Lowe, J., Chan, A., & Deneault, P. (1996a). Cost-benefit and cost-effectiveness analyses of behavioral marital therapy as an addition to outpatient alcoholism treatment. *Journal of Substance Abuse, 8,* 145-166.

O'Farrell, T. J., Choquette, K. A., Cutter, H. S. G., Brown, E. D., Bayog, R., McCourt, W., Lowe, J., Chan, A., & Deneault, P. (1996b). Cost-benefit and cost-effectiveness analyses of behavioral marital therapy with and without relapse prevention sessions for alcoholics and their spouses. *Behavior Therapy, 27,* 7-24.

O'Farrell, T. J., Cutter, H. S. G., Choquette, K. A., Floyd, F. J., & Bayog, R. D. (1992). Behavioral marital therapy for male alcoholics: Marital and drinking adjustment during the two years after treatment. *Behavior Therapy, 23,* 529-549.

O'Farrell, T. J. & Fals-Stewart, W. (2006). *Behavioral couples therapy for alcoholism and drug abuse.* New York: Guilford Press.

O'Farrell, T. J., & Fals-Stewart, W. (2001). Family-involved alcoholism treatment: An update. In M. Galanter (Ed.) *Recent developments in alcoholism, volume 15: Services research in the era of managed care* (pp. 329-356). New York: Plenum.

O'Farrell, T. J., & Murphy, C. M. (2002). Behavioral couples therapy for alcoholism and drug abuse: Encountering the problem of domestic violence. In C. Wekerle & A. M. Wall (Eds.), *The violence and addiction equation: Theoretical and clinical issues in substance abuse and relationship violence* (pp. 293-303). New York NY: Brunner-Routledge.

O'Farrell, T. J., & Murphy, C. M. (1995). Marital violence before and after alcoholism treatment. *Journal of Consulting and Clinical Psychology, 63,* 256-262.

O'Farrell, T. J., Murphy, C. M., Stephen, S., Fals-Stewart, W., & Murphy, M. (2004). Partner violence before and after couples-based alcoholism treatment for male alcoholic patients: The role of treatment involvement and abstinence. *Journal of Consulting and Clinical Psychology, 72,* 202-217.

Rosenthal, R. (1991). *Meta-analytic procedures for social research* (Revised edition). Newbury Park, CA: Sage Publications.

Schumm, J. A., O'Farrell, T. J., Murphy, M., & Fals-Stewart, W. (2006, November). *Outcomes following behavioral couples therapy for couples in which both partners have alcoholism versus couples in which only one partner has alcoholism.* Poster presented at the Annual Meeting of the Association for the Advancement of Behavioral and Cognitive Therapies, Chicago.

Stanton, M. D., & Shadish, W. R. (1997). Outcome, attrition, and family-couple treatment for drug abuse: A meta-analysis and review of the controlled, comparative studies. *Psychological Bulletin, 122,* 170-191.

Winters, J., Fals-Stewart, W., O'Farrell, T. J., Birchler, G. R., & Kelley, M. L. (2002). Behavioral couples therapy for female substance-abusing patients: Effects on substance use and relationship adjustment. *Journal of Consulting and Clinical Psychology, 70,* 344-355.

doi:10.1300/J020v26n01_10

A PRACTITIONER'S RESPONSE

Grace Happens

David C. Treadway, PhD

SUMMARY. Treatment models are important. The person and commitment of the therapist are even more important. doi:10.1300/J020v26n01_11 *[Article copies available for a fee from The Haworth Document Delivery Service: 1-800-HAWORTH. E-mail address: <docdelivery@haworthpress.com> Website: <http://www.HaworthPress.com> © 2008 by The Haworth Press. All rights reserved.]*

KEYWORDS. Alcohol and other drug use, treatment, models

David Treadway is in private practice in Weston, MA. His book, *Before It's Too Late: Working With Substance Abuse in the Family* (W.W. Norton, 1989) is a classic in the field of family-based treatment. *Intimacy, Change, and Other Therapeutic Mysteries: Stories of Clinicians and Clients* (Guilford, 2004) is intended to stimulate self-reflection among all practitioners, and the clients they serve.

[Haworth co-indexing entry note]: "Grace Happens." Treadway, David C. Co-published simultaneously in *Alcoholism Treatment Quarterly* (The Haworth Press) Vol. 26, No. 1/2, 2008, pp. 221-225; and: *Family Intervention in Substance Abuse: Current Best Practices* (ed: Oliver J. Morgan, and Cheryl H. Litzke) The Haworth Press, 2008, pp. 221-225. Single or multiple copies of this article are available for a fee from The Haworth Document Delivery Service [1-800-HAWORTH, 9:00 a.m. - 5:00 p.m. (EST). E-mail address: docdelivery@haworthpress.com].

Available online at http://atq.haworthpress.com
© 2008 by The Haworth Press. All rights reserved.
doi:10.1300/J020v26n01_11

INTRODUCTION

There is a softening in the air, a hint of spring. The night sky is lightening in the east. I've just finished reading this extraordinary collection of manuscripts. I feel a rush of delight and satisfaction because the authors on these pages have done their homework, researched their techniques, simplified their treatment protocols. They have developed truly systematic, reliable tools for navigating the dangerous shoals and impenetrable fogs of the alcoholic family system. I have spent my life sailing along this treacherous shore, feeling my way. I know these waters well. I have learned through a lifetime of trial and error. These authors are offering you a rich variety of state of the art radar, GPS, and depth finders, all the necessary instruments for the seasoned as well as the inexperienced explorer.

And I am worried about Kevin. He's missing since yesterday. Chris can't find him. He disappeared yesterday in a drunken rage. He could be holed up drinking in a bar. He could be passed out on the side of the road. He could be dead.

I met Kevin and Chris when he was 22 and she 21. They were newly-weds. They came from ferociously dysfunctional and alcoholic families. They were incredibly stressed because they were also parenting Kevin's three younger siblings whom he had taken in after the death of parents. Back then Kevin was very careful about his use of alcohol and Chris didn't drink at all. They were both so scared of that "evil stuff" as Chris would call it.

I worked with them for a few months and they did well and went on their way. A few years later, they came back because Kevin's drinking had evolved into alcoholism and Chris had evolved into the over-functioning, nagging spouse. We worked together again. Classic interventions of helping Chris disengage, and shifting the locus of responsibility onto Kevin's shoulders worked. I was privileged to attend his 1st anniversary A.A. celebration.

Chris got pregnant and they graduated again. Five years later they were included in my own follow up study. Clients I had seen at least five or more years previously were interviewed about their results from therapy; they were also assessed by the interviewer and then I was interviewed on my recollections of the therapy. The results were startling. There was very little correlation between my clinician's observations, my recollections, and those of the people I treated. Some people that I felt I had failed with credited me with having saved their family although to the interviewer that family appeared to still be in terrible shape. Other folks that I thought had done a great job, couldn't remember our work at all, and credited starting church back then as the reason why their family had made such dramatic progress.

The piece de resistance was one young college woman, whom I really liked and met with most of her freshman year, who could only remember meeting me once or twice, and couldn't recall anything about the encounter. But just as the researcher was turning off the tape, she said, brightly, "Oh, wait, I do remember something. One night, he walked me to my car because it was dark and the parking lot lights were out. And on the way, he said something that changed my life."

"My researcher asked, "What was that?"
"Oh, gee, I don't remember."

And when my interviewer asked me, I didn't even remember the walk to the car.

Kevin and Chris, and I, however, felt the same way about our experience. Kevin was still sober. He said, "Treadway brought us up."

I said, "I kind of adopted them."

They were one of my favorite success stories.

Then two years ago, Chris called me. "You're the only one that can straighten the lughead out. Will you take us back after all these years?"

By this time their older daughter was 22 and their younger was 19. Kevin turned 50. A lot of beer had flowed under the bridge. In these last couple of years, I've thrown some variation of many family therapy strategies mentioned in this book at them, Networking, Motivational Interviewing, Voluntary Intervention, CRAFT strategies, in particular. Despite brief glimpses of sobriety and sometimes successful controlled drinking, we were moving inexorably toward Chris insisting on a separation and me doing a therapeutic discharge. This is when I refuse to continue any treatment unless he goes into treatment. This is always a last step intervention that comes when the therapy itself can be seen as enabling the addiction and hopefully the possibility of terminating the therapy relationship carries some real weight with the client. I dreaded having to do it.

With Kevin, this slowly deteriorating situation was leading him toward desperation and suicidal despair, not recovery.

I felt as overwhelmed, helpless, and incompetent as I did when I started in the field 35 years ago. And that's the nature of the work with substance abusing family systems. They are often teetering on the edge of life and death, demanding effective intervention, but resisting everything we clinicians try to do. We are often treating multi-generational substance abuse in which the family that feuds together over drinking is often the family that sticks together with the drinking. The rest of the family is as entrenched in their patterned roles as the addict is. Hard nuts to crack. It is why the treatment models you have just read are so critically important. Most of the authors and myself have been promoting the value of family treatment of substance abuse for decades, but the outstanding contribution of these papers is that they establish the efficacy of family treatment. It works. It's cost effective. And teachable. These articles provide clear coherent models to train clinicians who too often are simply overwhelmed by the complexity, collusion, and crises of the alcoholic family.

But no matter how well thought out and articulated a treatment model may be, there is the one ingredient that is key to working well with these very difficult families: the person of the therapist. These families need therapists who will go the extra mile, or ten, or twenty. They need therapists who are unafraid to be lied to, blamed, and rejected. Therapists who dare to care. Dare to hope.

It's these personal qualities of the clinicians that come through the case reporting throughout these chapters. It's not simply the well designed interventions; it's the person of the therapist.

The following few paragraphs that I have distilled from my writing for thirty years really summarize the heart of the matter.

Treatment models are simply reference points that allow us generally to know where we are and where we are headed. The actual treatment is the process of integrating what we see in the family and the model we are using. The model helps us organize the data, pick out what is significant, anticipate responses, and to know which steps might be appropriate next. It is an organizational tool, a way of helping us think about our clients, ourselves, and the course of treatment.

However, we therapists practice an arcane art while feeling the weight of the expectation that we should be scientific and objective. No wonder many of us wonder if we are frauds or hypocrites. Yet we know, the map is not the territory and the model is not the treatment. After all the theories are spoken, and all of the therapeutic strategies applied, ultimately, what we have to offer our clients is our own flawed humanity and caring without shame. We are not all-knowing guides, marching fearlessly ahead of our clients as we lead them along the harrowing mountain trails. Yes, we do have pitons, ropes, and hammers. Yes, many of us have made the climb before. We have maps and weather reports. It is good to have experience and equipment. But, in the end, our willingness to share the risk, to give gentle voice to the fear, and to hold the sweaty palms is the gift that heals.

At least that's how it feels on the good days. On the bad days, we can feel like we're not much more than a "rent-a-friend," offering a less reliable result than your average escort service.

What happens in therapy may be a mystery. But, we, therapists, aren't. We are people with a calling: people who risk opening our hearts to the suffering of others. We believe that being one caring person, in one session, even one moment can sometimes be the difference that makes a difference.

It turns out Kevin wasn't passed out or dead. He was in jail. He drove himself off the road. He doesn't know whether it was a suicide attempt or not. Now he's scared out of his mind that he's going to be sentenced to serious jail time. And he's seriously sober, going to A.A. every day, taking his meds. He has been given the gift of desperation. As he said on the phone the other day, "I feel like whether I go to jail or not, I won't pick up again. Somehow my Higher Power let me live. I can't go back. After all these years, I really have hit my bottom."

I could hear it in his voice. I believe he's going to make it.

But if he does, it won't be my success story. And really not his either.

This is what I know:

If we dare to love,

Grace happens.

Sometimes.

Index